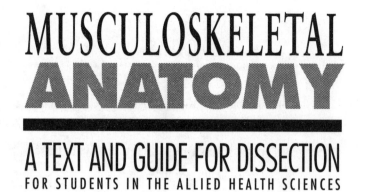

MUSCULOSKELETAL
ANATOMY

A TEXT AND GUIDE FOR DISSECTION
FOR STUDENTS IN THE ALLIED HEALTH SCIENCES

DEDICATION

This book is dedicated to those persons who have generously and selflessly donated their bodies for study by health science professionals. It is our hope that we may accomplish the goals of their trust, expressed by their bequests, in the delivery of sensitive and intelligently directed health care and education.

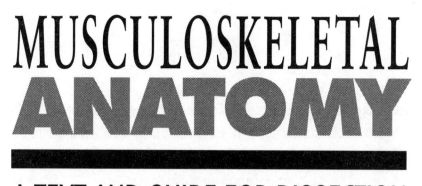

MUSCULOSKELETAL ANATOMY

A TEXT AND GUIDE FOR DISSECTION

FOR STUDENTS IN THE ALLIED HEALTH SCIENCES

Gene L. Colborn, Ph.D.

Professor of Anatomy
Department of Cellular Biology and Anatomy
Director, Center for Clinical Anatomy
Medical College of Georgia, Augusta, Georgia

David B. Lause, Ph.D.

Associate Professor and Course Director, Allied Health Anatomy
Department of Cellular Biology and Anatomy
Medical College of Georgia, Augusta, Georgia

The Parthenon Publishing Group

International Publishers in Medicine, Science & Technology

New York   London

Published in the USA by
The Parthenon Publishing Group Inc.
One Blue Hill Plaza,
PO Box 1564, Pearl River,
New York 10965

Published in Europe by
The Parthenon Publishing Group Limited
Casterton Hall, Carnforth,
Lancs LA6 2LA, UK

Library of Congress Cataloging-in-Publication Data

Colborn, Gene L.
    Musculoskeletal anatomy : a text and guide to dissection / Gene L. Colborn,
David B. Lause.
        p.   cm.
    Includes index.
    ISBN 1-85070-523-2 : $19.95
    1. Musculoskeletal system–Anatomy. 2. Musculoskeletal system–Dissection–
Laboratory manuals. I. Lause, David B. II. Title.
    [DNLM: 1. Musculoskeletal System–anatomy & histology–handbooks.
2. Dissection–handbooks. WE 39 C684m 1993]
QM100.C65 1993
611' .7'078–dc20
DNLM/DLC
for Library of Congress   93-13736
                                                                                    CIP

This edition published 1993

Printed in the United States

TABLE OF CONTENTS

PREFACE

Due to the rapid expansion of information in the biomedical sciences, and increasing sophistication in the treatment and care of patients, additional responsibilities are being placed on allied health professionals. It is somewhat disturbing that, at a time when there is continuing pressure to reduce the information load taught in basic science courses there is, paradoxically, a conflicting demand for students to know more clinically pertinent anatomy than ever before. Advances in biomedical engineering, electronic instumentation and analysis often require highly detailed knowledge of what in former days were considerd "minutiae."

In recent years, there have been significant changes in the philosophy underlying the teaching of gross anatomy. In many health science institutions, the classical gross anatomy course has been reoriented toward the teaching of clinically relevant anatomy. With this more practical approach, the basic facts are taught with a distinct emphasis upon providing information pertinent to clinical problem solving. It has been with this spirit that this book was conceived.

Musculoskeletal Anatomy is intended primarily to be a guide for the dissection of the back and limbs - regions which are specifically relevant in the education of students of occupational and physical therapy. It also contains data pertinent to many of the structures which are to be examined in the gross anatomy laboratory. Its instructional and didactic contents are supplemented by questions and answers, organized conveniently at the end of each chapter, which the student can use for self-assessment or review. The questions contain many of the fundamentals, the "essential" facts, which students are expected to learn in the typical program in anatomy. Clinical "pearls" are added often to illustrate the relevance of the facts to real life.

The vocabulary of gross human anatomy is both broad and rich. Unfortunately, much of its language is essentially unknown to the beginning student of the subject. For this reason, a list of definitions can be found at the end of each chapter, which may shed light upon some of the terms used in the preceeding pages.

There is a strong tendency for students to learn to identify structures in the laboratory and to memorize didactic material as though these are totally different tasks, each an end to itself. This text is intended to assist the student toward integration of the laboratory experience with that which is more "cerebral," so that each can reinforce the other and make for both easier recall and greater understanding.

This book is not intended to be a complete sourcebook of the functional anatomy of the musculoskeletal system. Its study should be accompanied by reference to a good pictorial atlas, both in the laboratory and in private. The student is encouraged to expand upon the information in this text/dissector by consulting one of the excellent textbooks of anatomy which are available.

IN MEMORIAM

Our Father, we know that we begin in the warm and watery darkness of our mother's womb. And all of us were pushed and pulled into the light of day. We have grown up in the light and we love the light. In the common light of day, we have found joy, knowledge, friends, pain and sorrow. It is all ours. And we would not leave even the sorrows of the light for the darkness of death. Yet, we move at death into the darkness and into another birth into eternal light. Have pity on us for our fear. We fear death because it dissolves the unity of the mind and the body and the destruction of our unity with our friends and lovers. We need the hope of a new unity of life beyond the darkness of death.

These persons we honor today, whose ashes are to be buried, gave their bodies to us for our learning. The greatest gift in human life is always the gift of self. In the trust of hands joined and of bodies pressed together, of persons united in the joy of friendship, of the sharing of all the gifts of human mind and body there is the gift of the human self.

So in giving the body after death, surely these persons gave something of themselves to us. If only an empty shell, as we might pick one off the beach and turn it over in our hands; so have we turned these bodies in our hands, seen their beauty of structure and have traced the handiwork of God.

We have learned also in touching these bodies something about death. Once they laughed, cried, fought and loved. And no longer do. They have spoken to us of our death and thus of all that human life contains. Let us remember from this, the depths each human life contains.

Let them rest in peace, may they forever walk in light. Amen.

A prayer offered during a student memorial service for body donors,
by the Reverend Joseph W. O'Brian, Spring, 1976

ACKNOWLEDGMENTS

The preparation of this book in its first edition (1989) was expedited by the expert assistance and hard work of Mr. Gary Berlin, software engineer, and the tireless efforts of Ms. Andrea Taylor Jordan, who first typed the manuscript into the computer-based format. We express our sincere appreciation to both of these individuals. Many of the figures in the text have been modified and adapted from original work of Mr. John Hagan and Ms. Karen Waldo. The outstanding skills of these two individuals are well recognized within the demanding world of medical illustration. We express thanks also to Urban and Schwarzenberg, Medical Publishers, and to Mr. Braxton Mitchell, former president of the American division of Urban and Schwarzenberg, for their support of the initial production of the artwork.

We greatly appreciate the many helpful suggestions, criticisms and comments made by collegues and students in the evolution of this text. In this regard, Dr. Michael Barrett, Associate Professor of Cellular Biology and Anatomy, and a dedicated instructor of Allied Health students has been of great help in filtering out textual and typographical errors. For those errors which remain within the text (factual and grammatical), we apologize and ask that you bring them to our attention for correction in the future.

Several invaluable resources were drawn upon in creating the lists of Definitions found at the end of each chapter in the textbook. We would like to acknowledge each of these superb dictionaries and an entertaining, as well as informative, etymologic sourcebook:

The Origin of Medical Terms by H.A. Skinner, Hafner Publishing Company, New York, 1970.
Stedman's Medical Dictionary, 24th Edition, Williams and Wilkins Publishing Company, Baltimore, 1982.
Dorland's Illustrated Medical Dictionary, 26th Edition, W.B. Saunders Company, Philadelphia, 1981.

Gene L. Colborn, Ph.D.
David B. Lause, Ph.D.
Augusta, Georgia, 1993

PART I

INTRODUCTION

CHAPTER 1: GENERAL ANATOMY

CHAPTER 1

GENERAL ANATOMY

Basic Terminology

Anatomical Nomenclature. Nomenclature is, essentially, the systematic naming of things (from the Latin *nomen* + *calare* = to call). The nomenclature of anatomy has a long and colorful history. In the past, over 50,000 anatomical terms were in use internationally to name the parts of the body, often with numerous terms applied to the same structure.

In 1895 the German Anatomical Society met in Basle and devised the Basle Nomina Anatomica (BNA), a list of some 5,000 words, to replace the confusing, often contradictory terminology which had developed in the scientific world to that time. The Commission set forth guidelines for the devising of names for anatomic structures, as follows:

1. With few exceptions, there should be only one name for each structure.

2. All names should be in Latin for international use.

3. The names of structures should be aids for memorization; that is, each term should have some informative or descriptive value.

4. Each term should be as brief and simple as possible.

5. Structures which are related topographically should have similar names (such as femoral nerve, femoral artery, femoral vein).

6. There should be usage of adjectives as opposites (for examples: pectoralis major, pectoralis minor; flexor digitorum superficialis and profundus; medial, lateral).

7. There should be no changes in familiar terms for purely pedantic reasons.

8. Eponyms should be discarded. Eponyms are names associated with persons, such as "Hunter's canal" for the adductor canal; "Poupart's ligament" for the inguinal ligament.

Revisions and corrections of the Nomina Anatomica have been made periodically during the twentieth century to make the language of anatomy truly international. In actual usage the Latin terminology of the Nomina Anatomica is often translated or transliterated to some degree into the language of the country wherein it is employed to facilitate understanding.

You will become aware of outmoded terms which are still used by anatomists and clinicians who do not know of, or are resistant to changes in the nomenclature of anatomy. Note for examples, the use of "internal mammary artery" for the internal thoracic artery and "innominate" for the brachiocephalic artery. The term "innominate" (definition: having no name) is really inappropriate for a major blood vessel which does, as a matter of fact, have a name. Some terms in rather common use are simply wrong, such as "calvarium," used as the singular for the calvaria or skull cap, the plural for which is calvariae.

The Skin

Composition. The skin is composed of two layers, the epidermis and the dermis (Fig. 1:1). The epidermis, the external layer of the skin, is derived embryologically principally from ectoderm. This outermost, cornified stratum of the skin is especially thick on the palms of the hands and the soles of the feet. It is very thin over the eyelids.

The dermis, or corium, is derived embryologically from mesenchyme; it is a strong layer of tough, fibrous connective tissue and it is rich in numbers of small blood vessels and nerves. This layer tends to be thicker on the extensor surfaces of the body such as the back, thinner on the flexor surfaces.

Fibrous bands, or strands, called **retinacula cutis** pass from the deep aspect of the corium into, and through the subcutaneous fat to attach the skin to underlying deep fascia. Compare the mobility of the skin of the palmar surfaces of your hands with that of the skin on the backs of your hands. The difference is, in part, a reflection of the presence or absence of the retinacula cutis. The retinacula cutis of the breast tissues, referred to clinically as the "suspensory ligaments" of the breast, may become contracted in breast cancer, resulting in a dimpling of the skin overlying a tumor. The dimpling provides a useful diagnostic aid to detection of the disease process.

Smooth muscle bundles, called **pilomotor muscles** (arrector pili) are present in the dermis

4

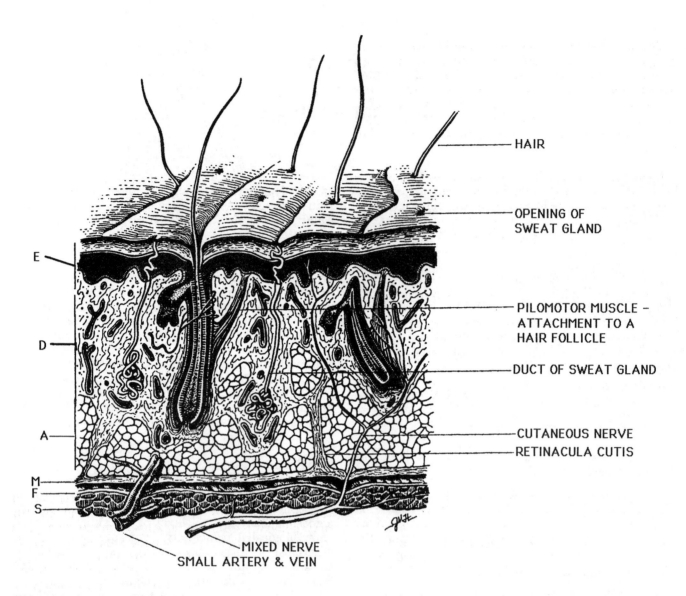

Figure 1:1 Skin and underlying fascial layers. E, epidermis; D, dermis; A adipose layer of subcutaneous tissue; M, membranous layer of subcutaneous tissue; F, deep fascia overlying skeletal muscle; S, skeletal muscle.

(Fig. 1:1). Such muscles attach to the undersurface of hair follicles. The pilomotor muscles are supplied by sympathetic autonomic nerve fibers. When stimulated to contract, these muscles cause elevation of the hairs (as in "goosebumps").

Glands of the Skin. Sebaceous glands secrete greasy sebum. These glands are situated within the dermis and are found frequently in hairy skin. The duct of a sebaceous gland usually ends at the side of an adjacent hair follicle. Some sebaceous glands are present in the dermis of the face; blockage of their ducts, with infection, results in acne.

Sweat glands are located adjacent to the deep surface of the dermis in hairy or hairless skin. The sweat gland ducts pass outward through the dermis and epidermis to empty upon the surface of the skin.

The openings of these glands can be seen easily with a low power magnifying lens.

Embryologic Derivatives of the Epidermis. Hairs grow from epithelial follicles, which are downgrowths of the epidermis. Hair is more plentiful upon the extensor surfaces of the limbs than upon the flexor surfaces. Nails develop from the epidermis. Sweat glands, sebaceous glands and the glandular elements of the mammary gland (breast) develop as downgrowths from the epidermis into, and through the dermis into the underlying fatty tissue.

Skin Creases and Lines of Cleavage of the Skin. The skin overlying the flexor surface of some joints is bound firmly to underlying structures such as deep fascia - creating the flexion creases. Note the palmar surfaces of the joints of your fingers and your wrists for examples of such creases.

5

Collagen bundles of the dermis tend to be arranged in parallel, creating **cleavage lines** in the skin known as the **lines of Langer** (Fig. 1:2). Where flexion creases are apparent, it can be assumed that the cleavage lines run parallel with them. The cleavage lines of the skin tend to pass circumferentially around the neck and trunk, but longitudinally in the limbs.

Incisions made parallel with the lines of cleavage heal with much less scarring and contracture than incisions made at right angles to the cleavage lines. This fact is especially important in cosmetic surgery, surgery of the hand and incisions in the abdominal wall.

Functions of the Skin. Forming nearly one-fifth of the weight of the body, the skin is one of the largest organs in the body, and performs a variety of functions - some obvious, and some not so obvious. The skin acts in the **conservation of body fluid**. The significance of this function is of special importance in burn patients.

The skin participates in the **regulation of body temperature** by acting as an insulator - together with the underlying subcutaneous tissues - by sweating, by insensible perspiration (diffusion of body fluid through the skin) and by neurovascular reflexes of cutaneous blood vessels.

The skin provides **good frictional properties for locomotion and manipulation.** It also acts in protection of the body against injury, invasion by microorganisms, etc. **Sensory perception** of the environment is provided by various somatic sensory nerve endings in the skin. It functions somewhat as an **excretory** and **absorptive** organ, and is important in the **formation of Vitamin D** in response to ultraviolet light.

"Referral" of pain to the skin of the surface of the body from an internal organ such as the heart is an important feature of many clinical diagnoses, although the mechanism of such referral is poorly understood. "Body language" is conveyed in part by almost subliminally perceived things such as skin coloration from vascular changes which occur in emotional states. Changes in the normal color, texture, temperature and moistness of the skin are often of diagnostic importance.

Fascia

Superficial Fascia. The superficial fascia is also called tela subcutanea, subcutaneous tissue, and the hypodermis (as in hypodermic needle). This is a layer of connective tissues which, among other things, serves in attaching the skin to underlying bone, deep fascia or muscular fascia by means of retinacula cutis. In certain parts of the body the superficial fascia is composed of an outer, fatty layer and a deeper, membranous layer. This is particularly

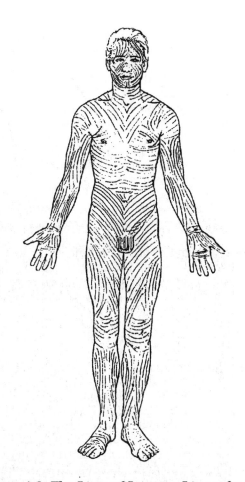

Figure 1:2 The Lines of Langer. Lines of tension, or cleavage lines, are produced in the skin by the arrangement of collagen bundles in the dermis. In a general way, the lines of tension tend to be roughly horizontal in arrangement in the skin of the trunk; they are more vertically aligned in the limbs. Incisions made parallel with these lines heal with less tendency to gap widely and heal with less scarring than incisions made at right angles to them.

true in the abdominal wall and in the proximal parts of the limbs. The fibrous and areolar tissues of the superficial fascia vary in their quantity of adipose tissue (fat) from one part of the body to another. There is little fat in the eyelids, for example, but the deposits in the buttocks, abdominal wall and limbs can be very great.

The superficial fascia contains thin muscles in some areas such as the neck, face, scalp and palms -muscles which insert into, and act to move the skin. The platysma muscle of the neck and the palmaris brevis muscle of the palm of the hand are examples of such muscles. Such subcutaneous muscles are distributed much more extensively in some lower mammals (in which it is called the panniculus carnosus), imparting to the animals considerable ability to move the skin rather freely.

6

Deep Fascia. The deep fascia is a variably thick, fibrous layer of connective tissue which lies deep to the superficial fascia, investing the muscles of the limbs and the body wall. This fascia is thickened in some parts of the body to form sites of attachment for the origins or insertions of skeletal muscles, and is often continuous with the connective tissue which invests most muscles. In addition, the limbs are divided into muscle compartments by the attachment of deep fascial septae (plural of septum: partitions) to bones.

The deep fascia takes the form of more or less distinct connective tissue partitions in certain areas of the body which assume clinical importance when they direct the spread of fluids, infectious processes and tumors from one area to another. Visceral fascia, such as that which separates the trachea and the pharynx in the neck, is often very significant in this role.

Muscle

General Characteristics. The musculature of the body can be categorized histologically and functionally as striated skeletal muscle, smooth muscle and cardiac muscle (Fig. 1:3). **Skeletal muscles**, also called somatic muscles, form the bulk of the musculature of the body. These are usually described in terms of their bony attachments (origins and insertions), functions and source of voluntary nerve supply.

Smooth muscle forms much of the substance of the walls of hollow organs and viscera of the body; it is present in blood vessels, larger lymphatic vessels and the pilomotor muscles of the dermis. Such muscle is innervated by autonomic or involuntary nerve fibers. **Cardiac muscle** is regulated, like smooth muscle, by autonomic nerves, but in the heart these nerves act to modulate the activity of intrinsic pacemaking and conducting cells which are specialized heart muscle cells.

Skeletal or Somatic Muscles. The individual skeletal muscles are characterized by their shape, their attachments, their functions and their specific nerve supply. All skeletal muscles are composed of individual contractile cells which are arranged either parallel with, or at oblique angles to the line of pull of the entire muscle (Fig. 1:4). The muscles which are composed principally of parallel fibers produce a greater range of movement of the part of the body moved, whereas muscles which are composed of oblique muscle fibers sacrifice range of movement for the capability of exerting greater strength of pull.

Muscles formed primarily of parallel fibers may be short and flat, straplike, or fusiform in overall appearance - such as the rhomboideus minor, sartorius and biceps brachii muscles, respectively. Muscles which are formed by oblique fibers are said to possess a pennate, semipennate or multipennate appearance - such as the rectus femoris, flexor pollicis longus and deltoid, respectively. The term "pennate" refers to the similarity of arrangement of the muscle fibers to the barbs of a feather.

Skeletal muscles are typically attached at both ends to bone by strong connective tissue fibers organized into **tendons**. Certain muscles, however, such as the muscles of facial expression, are attached at one end to skin rather than to bone. Tendons may have the form of cord-like, straplike or sheetlike condensations of connective tissue. The flattened tendons, such as that of the latissimus dorsi and certain of the abdominal muscles, are referred to as **aponeuroses** (singular: aponeurosis).

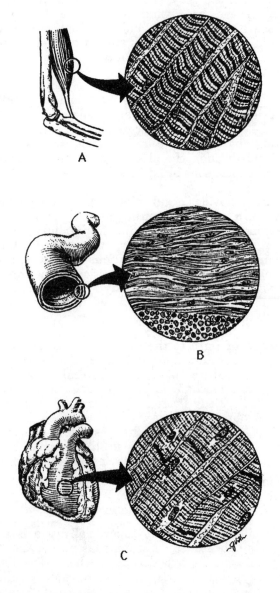

Figure 1:3 Contrasting histologic features of : A, skeletal muscle; B, smooth muscle; C, cardiac muscle.

7

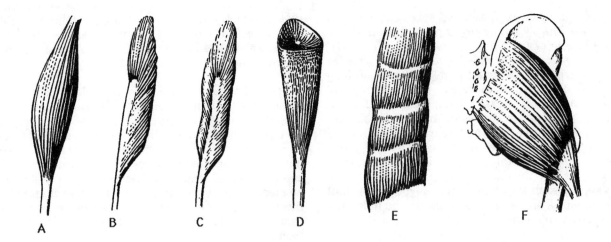

Figure 1:4 Variations in structure and form of skeletal muscle. A, fusiform muscle (ex., long head of biceps brachii); B, semipennate muscle (ex., flexor pollicis longus); C, pennate muscle (ex., rectus femoris); D, circumpennate muscle (ex., tibialis anterior); E, strap muscle(ex., rectus adbominis) and, F, quadrilateral muscle (ex., gluteus maximus).

The functions of skeletal muscles are governed chiefly by their specific sites of bony attachments; that is, their origins and insertions. Most skeletal muscles arise from a part of one bone and insert upon a part of another bone - in the process, crossing one or more joints between the two bones. The bony attachment which remains relatively fixed when the muscle contracts is called the **origin** of the muscle; that end which moves is designated as the **insertion** of the muscle.

The distinction between "origin" and "insertion" for some muscles is rather arbitrary. For instance, the insertion of the pectoralis major muscle of the chest wall is stated to be the humerus. The contraction of the muscle causes the arm to be drawn toward the chest because of the origin of the muscle from ribs, sternum and clavicle. If the arm is fixed in position, however, the pectoralis major can assist in breathing by drawing the ribs outward and upward. The origin and insertion of the muscle have therefore been reversed.

When a muscle contracts, it may do so as a **prime mover** at a joint between two bones. It may also function as a **synergistic muscle** with others in movement, as is often the case. A single muscle rarely acts alone as a prime mover, and its actions are influenced by the contraction or relaxation of other muscles. A muscle may also act to **stabilize** a joint, rather than to produce distinct joint movement; or it may function as an **antagonist** to other muscles acting upon a particular joint.

Bones and Joints

Functions of Bone. Bones provide support for the body. They are essential for producing postural, locomotive and manipulative actions in response to the contraction of skeletal muscles. Other important functions of bone include the formation of blood cells within the marrow of certain bones, calcium metabolism, and protection of softer, internal organs. Bone is a living tissue and, irrespective of its apparent rigidity and seeming inertness, has greater reparative capability than almost any other tissue of the body.

Periosteum. Bones are covered with a layer of tough, fibrous periosteum, except where they articulate in synovial joints (freely movable joints). The periosteum conveys blood vessels for the bone and provides cells for the formation of new bone, when called upon to do so. Periosteum is supplied richly by sensory fibers from the nerves of the overlying skin or from nerves which supply the muscles which lie adjacent to the bone; hence, injuries or disease processes affecting bone can be very painful,

Joints. Joints, or articulations, provide unions between bones. Joints can be immovable, slightly movable, or freely movable. Various systems of terminology have been devised to describe the numerous types of joints. Most such systems are rather confusing and inconsistent in application. Terms which are in use currently will be introduced later in the text, where it is appropriate to do so.

Some bones, such as those that form the vault of the skull, are simply joined together by fibrous tissue and are capable of little or no movement. Similarly, the junctions of bone and hyaline cartilage at **epiphyses** (regions of growth at the ends of long bones) and at the junctions of ribs with costal cartilages are also rather immobile. Limited movement is possible between bones which are covered at their ends by hyaline cartilage and joined together by dense fibrous tissue, such as the pubic symphysis and the intervertebral disks between vertebrae. Freely movable, or synovial joints are of several types, such as hinge joints, pivot joints, ball and socket joints and so on. All possess the following characteristics (illustrated in Fig. 1:5):

1. **The ends of the bones involved in the joint are covered with a layer of hyaline cartilage,** providing very smooth surfaces for movement.

2. **The ends of the articulating bones are joined together by a tough, fibrous articular capsule.**

3. **The fibrous capsule and the portions of the bones within the joint which are not in direct contact are covered with a membrane, the synovial membrane,** which secretes a slippery fluid for facilitation of movement between the bones.

The Cardiovascular System

The cardiovascular system consists of the heart, the blood vessels and lymphatic vessels. The general pattern of blood and lymphatic flow is described hereafter.

Blood-Vascular System. Deoxygenated blood is returned to the heart by the superior and inferior vena cavae. These two large veins terminate at the right atrium of the heart - the superior vena cava returning blood from the head, neck and upper limbs; the inferior vena cava returning venous blood from the lower limbs and abdominal area. [See figures1:7, 8.]

From the right atrium the blood from the body passes into the right ventricle and then into the pulmonary artery. This artery and its branches

distribute blood to the lungs, where gaseous exchange takes place. Freshly oxygenated blood is carried from the lungs to the left atrium of the heart by the pulmonary veins (Fig. 1:6, 7).

From the left atrium the blood flows into the left ventricle and then out of that chamber into the aorta. Major branches of the aorta and the peripheral arterial system then deliver blood to all parts of the body (Fig. 1:8). From the larger arteries the blood passes by small arterial branches and arterioles into capillary beds where exchange of gases, metabolic elements and fluid occurs. Small venules convey blood elements from the capillary beds to larger veins that ultimately transport the blood back again to the heart.

Arterial flow is directed initially by the contractile force exerted by the heart in systole. When the heart muscle relaxes in diastole the pulmonary and aortic valves prevent the arterial blood from flowing back again into the heart. The peripheral direction of flow of the arterial blood is assisted further by contractions of the muscular walls of the arteries.

The majority of the named arteries of the body are each accompanied by two or more veins which are applied closely to the arterial wall and which anastomose (communicate by collateral channels) with one another rather freely. When two or more veins accompany a single artery in this fashion they are referred to as the **venae comitantes** of the artery. In contrast to the arterial side of the blood-vascular system, the venous system is characterized by relatively low intravascular pressures. The additional channels provided by the venae comitantes assist in maximizing the rate of return of the venous blood to the heart.

Veins, in general, possess less smooth muscle in their walls than do their counterparts in the arterial system. Unidirectional flow in veins is assisted greatly by the presence of **valves**, particularly in the veins of the limbs. Contraction of skeletal muscles in the vicinity of veins causes compression of these vessels and thereby assists in moving the blood toward the heart. Differential pressures within the body cavities also participate in the regulation of the rates at which venous blood is returned to the heart.

The absence of valves in certain veins is clinically important in that the direction of flow within them can be reversed more readily. For example, infections in the face can spread in retrograde fashion to the brain by way of valveless veins which exist between these two regions.

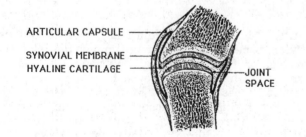

ARTICULAR CAPSULE
SYNOVIAL MEMBRANE
HYALINE CARTILAGE
JOINT SPACE

Figure 1:5 Characteristics of a typical synovial joint.

Lymphatic System. Most of the cells of the body are bathed in the fluid environment of the interstitial space (spaces between the cells). Certain large molecular weight substances that are present in the interstitial fluids are so large that they cannot pass freely into the capillaries of the blood-vascular system by diffusion or osmosis. These elements pass through openings in the walls of lymphatic capillaries, and are then carried as part of the lymph into increasingly larger lymphatic vessels.

Lymph is filtered in its passage through lymph nodes, and gradually concentrated by diffusive and osmotic processes. The terminal lymphatic vessels carry the lymph to large veins wherein the lymphatic elements mix with the blood. Much of the total volume of the lymph enters the venous system by way of large lymphatic vessels which join the internal jugular and subclavian veins at the root of the neck. The openings of these lymphatics into the large veins are guarded by unidirectional valves which ensure one-way flow of the lymphatic fluid and its contents into the venous blood.

The largest of the lymph vessels, the **thoracic duct**, begins in the upper abdominal region by the junction of several large tributaries; after passing upwards through the chest, it terminates at the junction of the left internal jugular vein and the left subclavian vein.

Although the larger lymphatic vessels possess smooth muscle in their walls, the flow of lymph is directed largely by the presence of valves throughout the lymph-vascular system - as was also seen to be the case in the venous system.

Efficient lymphatic flow is assisted greatly by the constrictive forces provided by the contraction of

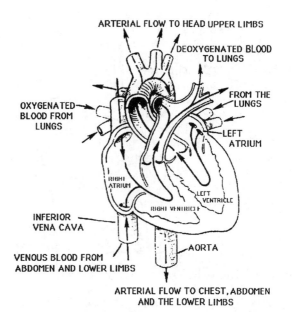

Figure 1:7 Blood flow to and from the heart. The vessels and chambers of the heart have been opened up to show the primary pathways of blood to and from the heart.

skeletal muscle within closed fascial compartments. If there is not enough muscle contraction, "pooling" of the lymph can occur locally. You have probably noticed the swelling that can take place in the feet and ankles when a person stands for a very extended period of time, especially if little or no muscular activity is occurring in the feet and legs at the time - as when one stands at attention.

The Nervous System

Composition. The nervous system can be divided conveniently into the central nervous system (CNS) and the peripheral nervous system (PNS). The central nervous system consists of the brain and the spinal cord; the peripheral nervous system is composed of the cranial nerves, nerve plexuses and ganglia.

The Neuron. The functional unit of the nervous system is the neuron (Fig. 1:9). A neuron is composed of a nerve **cell body** (or, soma) and its **processes**. The cell body of the neuron performs the metabolic activity necessary to the life of the neuron. Neuronal processes include dendrites and axons.

Generally speaking, a process or nerve fiber which carries an impulse toward the CNS or a nerve cell body is called a **dendrite** or **afferent fiber**. A process which carries an impulse away from the nerve cell body is called an **axon** or **efferent fiber**. Peripheral nerves can be composed almost entirely of fibers of one functional type - such as sensory, skeletal motor, or autonomic - or, as in mixed nerves,

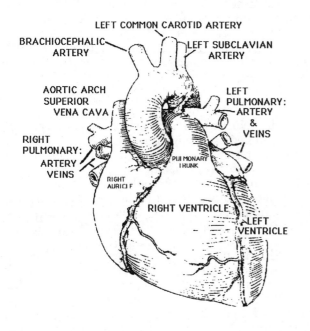

Figure 1:6 The heart and great vessels.

10

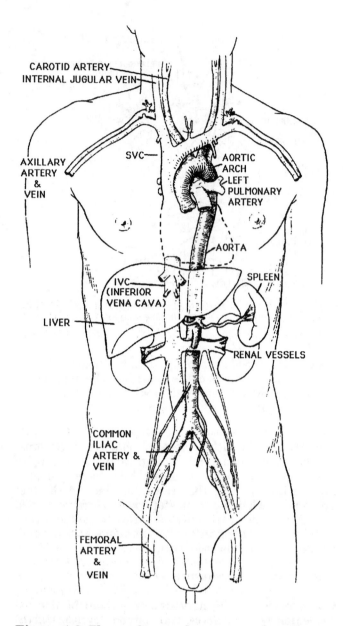

CAROTID ARTERY
INTERNAL JUGULAR VEIN

AXILLARY
ARTERY
&
VEIN

SVC

AORTIC
ARCH
LEFT
PULMONARY
ARTERY

AORTA

IVC
(INFERIOR
VENA CAVA)

SPLEEN

LIVER

RENAL VESSELS

COMMON
ILIAC
ARTERY &
VEIN

FEMORAL
ARTERY
&
VEIN

Figure 1:8 The cardiovascular system. Anterior view of some of the major arteries and veins. The position of the heart is indicated by the dotted line.

they can contain more than one of the various fiber types.

Some neuronal processes are very long; some are quite short. A dendrite carrying sensation all the way from the skin of a stubbed toe to the CNS, for example, is very long, indeed! Other processes, such as those which provide communication between adjacent neuronal cell bodies can be less than a millimeter long.

The neuron illustrated in Figure 1:9 represents an efferent or motor neuron. As will be seen later, other neurons differ markedly in appearance from that

illustrated - in shape, size and in arrangement of their processes.

Nerves. Nerves are constructed much like an electric cable composed of many individual wires, each insulated separately, and all bound together in a common sheath. Using this common analogy, nerves are composed of diverse numbers of processes of neurons held together by a common connective tissue sheath. Some nerves are no thicker than a hair; others, like the sciatic nerve of the lower limb, can be more than a centimeter in diameter. Large nerves contain many thousands of neuronal processes or fibers, each of which is so small as to be seen only with the aid of a microscope.

Cranial and Spinal Nerves. Twelve pairs of nerves arise from the brain; these are called cranial nerves. They arise, more specifically, from the brainstem. The names of the twelve cranial nerves are listed in Table 1:1, together with a simple description of the primary function or functions of each nerve. Notice that the name of each cranial nerve is associated with a Roman numeral designation. These numerals are commonly used as synonyms for the anatomic names. (For example, "Bell's palsy", or paralysis of the muscles of facial expression, results from disorders of the seventh cranial nerve.)

Thirty-one pairs of spinal nerves arise segmentally from the spinal cord. Each spinal nerve (Fig. 1:10-12) is formed by the fusion of dorsal and ventral roots, each of which is composed of processes of many neurons. The dorsal roots carry sensory processes; the ventral roots carry motor axons. Each spinal nerve divides into a dorsal primary ramus which supplies tissues of the back, and a ventral primary ramus which supplies tissues of the limbs and ventral parts of the neck and body wall. The dorsal root ganglion on each dorsal root contains the cell bodies of all of the sensory fibers received by a given spinal nerve.

Nuclei. Nuclei are aggregations or collections of nerve cell bodies within the CNS; that is, within the brain or the spinal cord. This term should not be confused with the "nucleus" or "nuclei" found within most living cells. The oculomotor nucleus of the brain, for example, contains the cell bodies of axons which innervate muscles that move the eyeball. [Note that **nucleus** is singular; **nuclei** is plural.]

Ganglia. **Ganglia** are collections of nerve cell bodies outside of, or external to the CNS. Ganglia are often visible grossly as swellings upon individual cranial or spinal nerves or within nerve plexuses in the body cavities (such as the celiac and mesenteric plexuses of the abdomen). Certain ganglia are very small and can be seen only with the aid of some magnification or by microscopy. The cell bodies of some ganglia are scattered quite diffusely rather than in compact

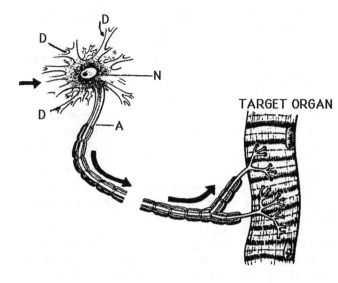

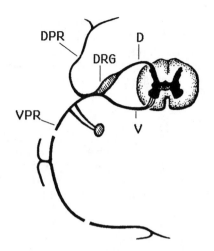

Figure 1:9 A neuron. In this example (a multipolar neuron), dendrites (D) are stimulated by other neurons in the central nervous system. From the cell body (N) the impulse is carried by an axon (A) to the target organ - here a skeletal muscle. The axon in this drawing is ensheathed segmentally by myelin, a lipid.

Figure 1:10 A "Typical" Spinal Nerve. (D) Dorsal root; (DPR) dorsal primary ramus; (DRG) dorsal root ganglion; (V) ventral root; (VPR) ventral primary ramus.

masses, as in the case of autonomic ganglia in the wall of the small intestine. [Note that **ganglion** is singular; **ganglia** is the plural form of this word.]

Types of Ganglia. Ganglia are either sensory or autonomic in function. **Sensory ganglia** are composed of cell bodies that possess a **peripheral process** which conveys information from a peripherally located receptor (such as a receptor for touch in the skin) to the ganglion, and a **central process** which carries the impulse into the brain or spinal cord for processing.

Sensory ganglia are paired structures; that is, each ganglion on one side of the body has a counterpart on the opposite (contralateral) side of the body. There are, for instance, 31 pairs of dorsal root ganglia associated with the paired spinal nerves near their attachment to the spinal cord. Paired sensory ganglia are also present in the head, and are characteristic features of certain of the cranial nerves.

Autonomic ganglia contain the cell bodies of neurons that innervate smooth muscle, cardiac muscle and glands. These ganglia are motor in function and are described typically as belonging either to the sympathetic division or the parasympathetic division of the autonomic nervous system (ANS) - described below.

All of the paired autonomic ganglia within the head, and the unpaired, diffuse terminal ganglia present upon, or near organs within the neck and

trunk are functional components of the parasympathetic division of the autonomic nervous system.

Bilateral "chains" of paravertebral ganglia in the neck and trunk and midline, prevertebral ganglia within the abdomen are important components of the sympathetic division of the autonomic nervous system. The paravertebral ganglionated chains are segmental in appearance, each one bearing a resemblance to a beaded necklace. The arrangement of the "beads" - each a ganglion - is that of one for each vertebral level bilaterally. In the cervical region (the neck), the arrangement is somewhat different, altered by fusion of adjacent ganglia in embryologic development.

The Autonomic Nervous System. The autonomic, or involuntary nervous system embodies elements both of the central and the peripheral parts of the nervous system. The autonomic nervous system consists of two major divisions, the sympathetic division and the parasympathetic division.

Sympathetic and parasympathetic neurons provide the efferent, or **motor**, nerve supply for **smooth muscle, cardiac muscle** and **glands.** In general terms, the two divisions have opposite effects upon the tissue or organ being supplied; for instance, parasympathetic fibers cause a decrease in heart rate and sympathetic fibers cause rate acceleration.

The sympathetic and parasympathetic systems utilize a **two-neuron pathway** in supplying smooth muscle, cardiac muscle or glands; that is, two neurons are arranged as in a series electrical hook-up between the CNS and the target to be innervated. The cell body of the first, or **primary neuron** (also referred to as the preganglionic neuron) is located within the brain or spinal cord. The **secondary neuron** (or, postganglionic neuron) is situated outside the CNS in an outlying autonomic ganglion.

Autonomic innervation takes place typically in the following way. First, the primary neuron is activated or stimulated by other neurons within the CNS. The axon of the primary neuron leaves the CNS and synapses (makes electrical or chemical contact) in an outlying autonomic ganglion with several or many secondary neuron cell bodies. The axons from these secondary cells then pass to the organs or cells supplied, stimulating or inhibiting their functions.

It has been estimated that some primary sympathetic axons can synapse with as many as two hundred secondary neurons. It is by recruitment of other neurons in such fashion that the activation of relatively few primary neurons can result in widely-spread effects throughout the body.

The Voluntary Nervous System. The voluntary nervous system provides the motor supply for skeletal, or somatic, muscles. The name for this system is somewhat misleading in that many individual skeletal muscles function without obvious, conscious thought. The muscular thoracic diaphragm - the principal respiratory muscle - contracts rhythmically without our thinking about it. The tiny skeletal muscles of the middle ear contract reflexively to sound without our directing them to do so. Likewise, when we move a limb or bend our backs or necks, it is not necessary for one to think about each individual muscle involved in a given movement; movements would otherwise be slow, indeed!

The cell bodies of skeletal motor neurons are located within various nuclei in the gray matter of the brain and spinal cord. The axons of these neurons leave the central nervous system within cranial or spinal nerves and are distributed by these to the skeletal muscles which they supply. Therefore, activation of a skeletal motor neuron ordinarily results in a very rapid, and specific initiation of contraction of muscle fibers. Those neurons which pass directly to skeletal muscle are referred to as **lower motor neurons**. Interruption of the axons of lower motor neurons or destruction of their cell bodies results in flaccid paralysis of the muscles which they supply.

Lower motor neurons can be excited by other neurons that have their cell bodies in the cerebral cortex, called **upper motor neurons**. Loss of upper motor neurons results in a spastic type of paralysis. Lower motor neurons can be caused to fire by impulses from other CNS neurons (such as fibers from the cerebellum, for example), or by sensory fibers from the periphery which synapse directly upon them. Interruption of CNS feedback circuits can lead to lack of muscular coordination. Abolition of reflexes such as the knee jerk occurs after interruption of sensory-motor reflex pathways.

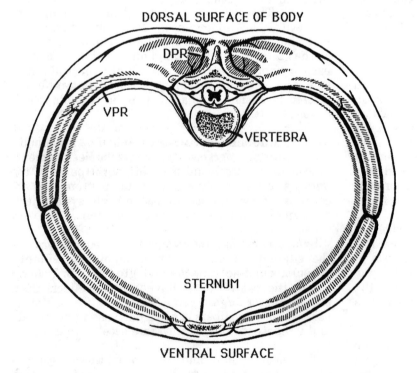

Figure 1:11 Distribution of a typical spinal nerve. From their origin within the spinal column, the spinal nerves emerge into the tissues of the body wall (and limbs). **DPR**, dorsal primary ramus; **VPR**, ventral primary ramus.

13

TABLE 1:1 THE CRANIAL NERVES

NERVE	PRINCIPAL FUNCTIONS
I OLFACTORY	Sense of smell
II OPTIC	Sense of vision
III OCULOMOTOR	Supplies five extraocular muscles and the pupillary constrictor of the eyeball.
IV TROCHLEAR	Supplies the superior oblique muscle of the eyeball
V TRIGEMINAL	Supplies the chewing muscles; primary sensory nerve of the head.
VI ABDUCENS	Supplies the lateral rectus muscle of the eyeball.
VII FACIAL	Supplies muscles of facial expression; sense of taste for anterior part of the tongue; supplies salivary glands with secretory fibers.
VIII VESTIBULOCOCHLEAR	Senses of hearing and equilbrium
IX GLOSSOPHARYNGEAL	Sensory supply of soft palate, pharynx; supplies the stylopharyngeus muscle.
X VAGUS	Supplies the muscles of the pharynx, larynx; provides para sympathetic fibers for the neck, chest and abdominal regions.
XI SPINAL ACCESSORY	Supplies the trapezius and sternocleidomastoid muscles
XII HYPOGLOSSAL	Supplies most muscles of the tongue.

The Anatomic Position and Anatomic Planes

Anatomic Position. For descriptive purposes the human body should be visualized in the "anatomic position," with the arms at the sides with palms facing forward and thumbs pointing laterally; the feet are together with the toes pointing forward, and the eyes are directed straight ahead (Figures 1:13, 14). This arbitrary, but useful convention is applied to the body to achieve uniformity of terminology, particularly in the use of terms describing the relations of body parts, such as "superior," "inferior," "medial," "lateral," the "radial side of the forearm," the "fibular side of the leg," and so on.

The usefulness of the concept of the anatomical position becomes quite apparent when one attempts to describe the relations of the parts of the body when they deviate from the normal. When you are reading the instructions for dissection, or studying a region of the body, you must imagine that the cadaver is in the anatomic position even though the body is lying prone or supine on the table, and the limbs are not straight - which is often the case.

Anatomic Planes. In descriptions of the body or its parts, frequent use is made of conventional anatomic planes (Figure 1:14).

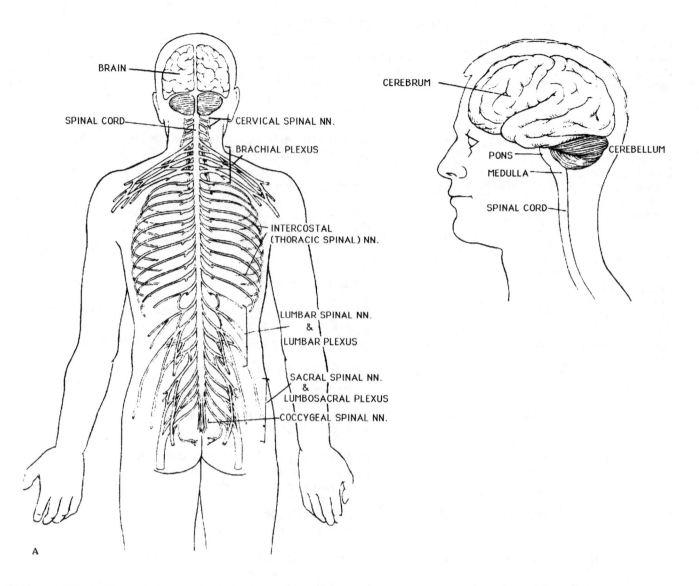

Figure 1:12 A, Dorsal view of the brain, spinal cord and the spinal nerves arising from the spinal cord. The brain and spinal cord form the central nervous system. The spinal nerves, the various nerve plexuses and ganglia form the peripheral nervous system. B, A lateral view of the brain and some of its subparts.

A **coronal** or **frontal plane** is one which divides the body or a body part into front (ventral) and back (dorsal) portions. A **sagittal plane** is a vertical plane which divides the body or a body part into right and left, or medial and lateral portions. A **mid-sagittal plane** is a longitudinal plane which divides a structure into equal parts; a **para-sagittal plane** is one which is parallel with, but to the side of, the mid-line or longitudinal axis. A **transverse or horizontal plane** is one which is perpendicular to the longitudinal axis of the body or a part of the body.

Terms of Movement

Several factors are involved in the diversity of types of movements which can occur at a given synovial joint. These factors include the shapes of the bony surfaces which are involved in the articulation, the structure of the associated ligaments, and the muscles which act upon the joint. Some of the terms used in describing joint movements are defined and illustrated hereafter with drawings of the upper limb (Fig. 1:15,21) - a part of the body normally possessing great mobility.

Flexion/Extension. In flexion (def.: a flexing or bending), the parts connected by a joint are brought closer together (Figs. 1:15,16). In flexion of the elbow, the arm and forearm are brought closer together. In extension, the parts connected by a joint are separated from one another or straightened. In

15

extension of the elbow, the arm and forearm are straightened out. Flexion of the spine results in a forward bending of the torso; extension straightens the spine. In plantar flexion of the foot, the foot or toes are directed downward; in dorsiflexion, the foot is turned upward.

Adduction/Abduction. In adduction (def.: to carry toward) a limb is brought toward the midline of the body. Adduction of a finger or toe brings it to the midline of the hand, or foot, respectively. Abduction (def.: to carry away from) is movement away from the midline (Fir. 1:17, 18).

Pronation/Supination. In pronation, the palm of the hand is caused to be turned dorsally (Fig. 1:19), and in supination the palm faces ventrally, as in the anatomic position. The body lies in the prone position when the ventral surface is directed downward; it is in the supine position when the ventral surface of the body is directed upward, as when you are lying on your back.

Rotation. Rotation is the turning of a structure around its axis. In the case of the upper limb, the arm can undergo limited medial or lateral rotation about the longitudinal axis of the humerus in the shoulder joint (Fig. 1:20).

Circumduction. Circumduction causes the distal portion of a body part - a limb, for example - to move in a circular direction (Fig. 1:21). Circumduction of the shoulder joint occurs when one draws a large circle on the wall. Notice in the example given that the finger tips would describe the base of a cone, the apex of which is located at the shoulder joint. This seemingly simple movement involves sequential combinations of abduction, adduction, flexion, extension and rotation at a joint.

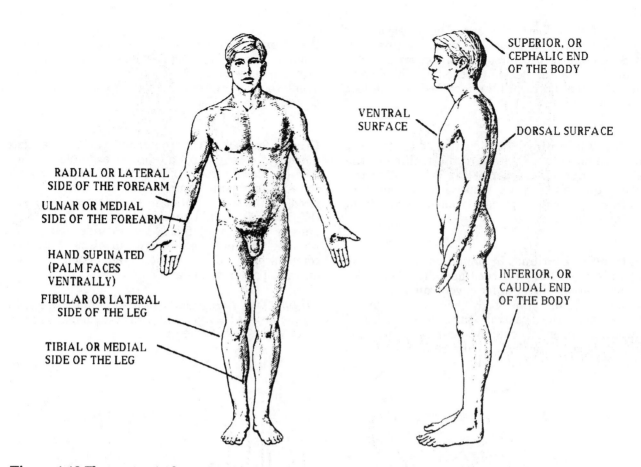

RADIAL OR LATERAL
SIDE OF THE FOREARM

ULNAR OR MEDIAL
SIDE OF THE FOREARM

HAND SUPINATED
(PALM FACES
VENTRALLY)

FIBULAR OR LATERAL
SIDE OF THE LEG

TIBIAL OR MEDIAL
SIDE OF THE LEG

SUPERIOR, OR
CEPHALIC END
OF THE BODY

VENTRAL
SURFACE

DORSAL SURFACE

INFERIOR, OR
CAUDAL END
OF THE BODY

Figure 1:13 The anatomical position - front and side views.

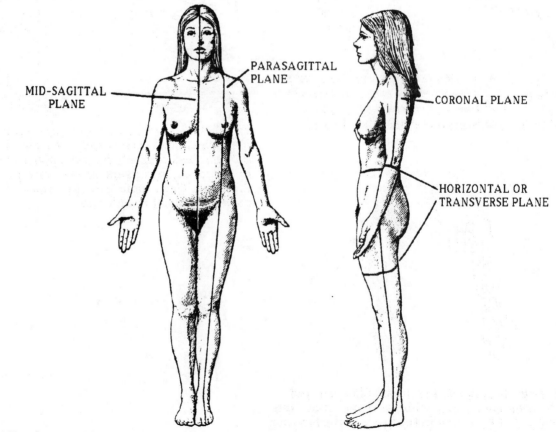

MID-SAGITTAL
PLANE

PARASAGITTAL
PLANE

CORONAL PLANE

HORIZONTAL OR
TRANSVERSE PLANE

Figure 1:14 Fundamental anatomic planes - frontal and lateral views.

17

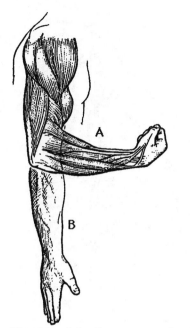

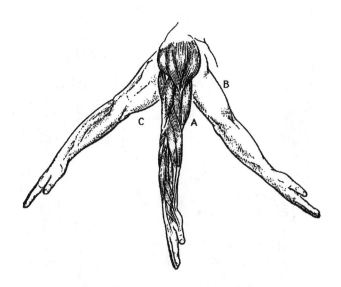

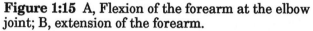

Figure 1:15 A, Flexion of the forearm at the elbow joint; B, extension of the forearm.

Figure 1:16 A, anatomic position of limb; B, flexion of the arm at the shoulder joint; C, extension of the arm at the shoulder joint.

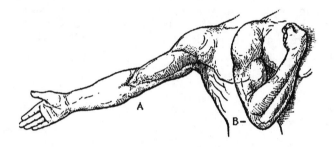

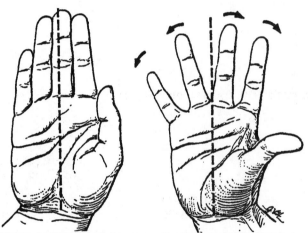

Figure 1:17 A, Abduction of the arm at the shoulder joint,with the elbow extended; B, arm adducted at the shoulder joint and rotated medially (inwardly) somewhat;the elbow,wrist and digits are flexed.

Figure 1:18 In abduction, the fingers move away from the midline of the hand (dotted line) and the thumb moves ventrally from the plane of the palm. In adduction, the fingers move toward the midline of the hand . The thumb is drawn toward the side of the palm when it is adducted.

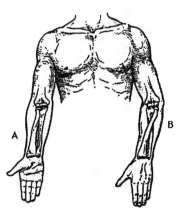

Figure 1:19 A, supinated position of forearm and hand; B, pronated position of forearm and hand. Note the change in the position in the bones of the forearm.

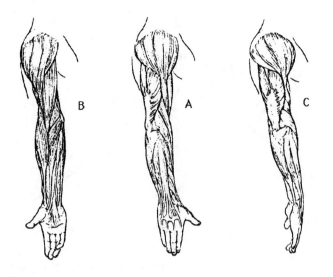

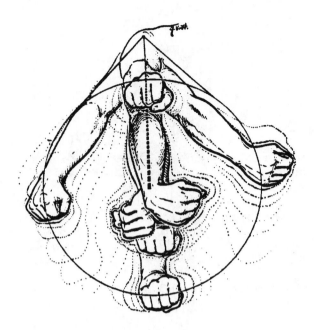

Figure 1:20 Rotation of arm at shoulder joint. At A, the arm is intermediate in position - between full lateral rotation at B and medial rotation at C.

Figure 1:21 Circumduction. The movement of the distal end of the limb (here, the hand) to describe a circle is called circumduction. The movement of a body part about its long axis (note the dotted line passing up the limb) is rotation. The latter should not be confused with the movements seen in pronation and supination - which involves the elbow and wrist joints.

Questions for review and study

1. _____ are strands of connective tissue that arise from the dermis and assist in binding the skin to underlying tissue.

Retinacula cutis

2. _____ insert upon hairs and cause their elevation, producing "gooseflesh."

Pilomotor muscles

3. From what layer of skin do sweat glands and the mammary gland develop embryonically?

The epidermis

4. What are the "lines of Langer?"

The lines of Langer, or cleavage lines of the skin, are lines of tension produced by the arrangement of collagen fibers in the dermis. The orientation of these lines often affects the placement of incisions, so that scarring can be reduced and the rate of healing accelerated.

5. Name the two layers of tissue that compose the superficial fascia in many parts of the body.

The adipose layer and the membranous layer

6. Name the layer of fascia that lies deep to the membranous layer of the tela subcutanea.

The deep, or muscular, fascia lies deep to the tela, or superficial fascia.

7. What three types of tissues receive their efferent (motor) supply from autonomic nerves?

Smooth muscle, cardiac muscle and glands

8. What type of tissue receives its efferent (motor) supply from voluntary or somatic nerves?

Skeletal, or somatic, muscle

9. _____ are flattened, sheet-like tendons.

Aponeuroses

10. The bony attachment of a muscle, which remains relatively stationary when a skeletal muscle contracts, is referred to as the _____ of that muscle.

The origin

11. The bony attachment of a muscle, which describes some range or degree of movement when the muscle contracts is referred to as the _____ of that muscle.

The insertion

12. What are the functions of skeletal muscle?

Skeletal muscles may act as: prime movers of a joint; synergists with other muscles in joint movements; stabilizers of a joint; antagonists to other muscles in movements of joints.

13. What are the three general functional types of articulations?

Articulations, or joints, can be immovable, slightly movable, freely movable.

14. What is the term that is applied to freely movable joints?

Synovial joints

15. What are the principal characteristics of a synovial joint?

a. The articulating bony surfaces are covered with hyaline cartilage.

b. The bones are held together by a fibrous articular capsule (which may be reinforced by ligaments).

c. The articular capsule is lined with a synovial membrane that secretes the lubricatory synovial fluid.

d. Some synovial joints contain a fibrous articular disk that may cushion the opposed ends of the bones, assist in spreading the synovial fluid within the joint, and increase the types of movement which can occur at the joint.

16. When two or more veins accompany a single artery they are referred to as_____.

Venae comitantes

17. What is an anastomosis?

An anastomosis is a direct communication between two vessels which can allow blood to flow freely between them in either direction. (Def.: from ana - through + stoma - a mouth) For example, the venae comitantes of an artery possess numerous anastomoses with one another.

18. What are the principal factors involved in the unidirectional flow of fluids within venous and lymphatic channels?

Unidirectional flow in veins and lymphatics is assisted by the presence of numerous valves, by the contraction of adjacent skeletal muscles, and by the changes of pressure within body cavities.

19. What is the CNS?

The central nervous system (CNS) consists of the brain and the spinal cord.

20. What is the peripheral nervous system?

The peripheral nervous system includes twelve pairs of cranial nerves, 31 pairs of spinal nerves, peripheral ganglia and nerve plexuses, and their derivatives.

21. What is a neuron?

A neuron consists of a nerve cell body and its processes, the dendrites and axon. The neuron is the functional unit of the nervous system.

22. What are efferent nerve fibers?

Motor nerve fibers. Motor fibers can be either autonomic or skeletal motor in function.

23. What are afferent nerve fibers?

Sensory fibers

24. What is a mixed nerve?

A mixed nerve contains motor and sensory fibers

25. What types of fibers are present in cutaneous nerves?

Cutaneous nerves contain sensory and postganglionic sympathetic nerve fibers.

26. What types of nerve fibers are present in a spinal nerve?

Spinal nerves contain sensory, autonomic and skeletal motor fibers.

27. What are nuclei?

Nuclei are collections or aggregations of nerve cell bodies in the CNS.

28 What are ganglia?

Ganglia are aggregations of nerve cell bodies in the peripheral nervous system.

29. What functional types of nerve cell bodies are present within ganglia?

A ganglion can consist of sensory or autonomic nerve cell bodies.

30. What structural type of neuronal cell body is found in a sensory ganglion?

The most common type of neuronal cell body in sensory ganglia is that which possesses a peripheral process which terminates in a sensory receptor and a central process which ends within the CNS. (Such neurons are called pseudounipolar neurons.)

31. What types of synapses (electrical connections between nerve cells) occur in sensory ganglia?

There are no synapses in sensory ganglia.

32. What types of nerve cell bodies are found in autonomic ganglia?

The cell bodies present in autonomic ganglia are secondary, or postganglionic in function; they are multipolar in structure.

33. What types of synapses are present in autonomic ganglia?

The processes (axons) of primary autonomic nerve cells synapse upon the cell bodies of secondary autonomic nerve cells in autonomic ganglia.

34. Where are the cell bodies of primary autonomic neurons found?

Primary, or preganglionic neuronal cell bodies are located within nuclei of the brain or spinal cord.

35. How long is the axon of a primary, or preganglionic neuron?

The axon of a preganglionic neuron continues to the ganglion wherein it synapses. An individual axon can pass through one or more ganglia before it synapses, but it is still referred to as "preganglionic" until it reaches its specific site of termination.

36. Where are the cell bodies of voluntary or skeletal motor neurons located?

Within nuclei of the CNS

37. What is the functional division of the ANS which functions in fight or flight responses?

The sympathetic division

38. What functional division of the autonomic nervous system is principally responsible for homeostatic responses?

The parasympathetic division

39. What is the position of the hands in the "anatomical position?"

The hands are supinated (palms facing ventrally) with the thumbs pointing laterally away from the body.

40. What kind of incision, anatomically, would pass down the midline of the abdominal wall?

A midsagittal incision

41. What kind of incision, anatomically, would pass vertically from the highest point of the skull to a point just in front of the ear?

A coronal incision

42. Describe the positions of the hands and their digits in the figures below, using the proper terms of movement.

In A, the wrist and fingers are extended and the thumb is adducted (flat against the side of the palm). In B, the wrist, fingers and thumb are in positions of flexion. Note that movements of the thumb occur in a plane which is perpendicular to that of movements of the fingers. (This will be discussed fully when the hand is studied.)

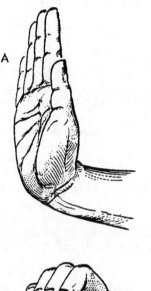

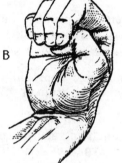

23

DEFINITIONS

Abduction [L. *ab* , from + *ducere,* to draw]
To draw away from the median plane or from the axial line of a limb.

Adduction [L. *ad,* to or toward + *ducere,* to draw toward]
To draw toward the median plane or toward the axial line of a limb.

Aponeurosis (pl. aponeuroses) [Gr. a tendon]
A white, flattened or ribbon-like tendinous expansion, serving mainly to connect a muscle with the parts that it moves.

Circumduction [L. *circumducere,* to draw around]
The active or passive circular movement of a limb or of the eye.

Epiphysis (epiphyses) [Gr. "an ongrowth"; excrescence]
The end of a long bone, usually wider than the shaft, and either entirely cartilaginous or separated from the shaft by a cartilaginous disk.

Extension [L. *extendo,* stretch out]
The movement by which the two ends of any jointed part are drawn away from each other.

Fascia (pl. fasciae) [L. "band"]
A sheet or band of fibrous tissue such as lies deep to the skin or forms an investment for muscles and various organs of the body.

Flexion [L. *flecto,* to bend]
The act of bending or condition of being bent.

Ganglion (pl. ganglia) [Gr. knot]
A general term for a group of nerve cell bodies located outside the central nervous system.

Innominate - Having no name.

Nomenclature [L. *nomen,* name + *calare,* to call]
A classified system of names.

Periosteum [Gr. *peri-* + *osteon* bone]
A specialized connective tissue covering all bones of the body and possessing bone-forming potential.

Pilomotor [L. *pilo-* + *motor,* move]
Pertaining to the arrector muscles the contraction of which produces cutis anserina (goose flesh) and the erection of the hairs.

Retinaculum (pl. retinacula) [L. "a rope, cable"]
A structure which retains an organ or tissue in place.

Supination [L. *supinus,* lying on the back; face upward]
Lying with the face upward.

Venae Comitantes – Accompanying veins of an artery.

PART II

THE BACK

CHAPTER 2

THE SKIN AND MUSCLES OF THE BACK

Note:

Read the entire chapter before attempting the dissection that follows. One can always run into unforeseen problems in a particular dissection and accidents can happen, but adequate preparation will make these less likely to occur. They are inevitable, otherwise.

A thorough knowledge of superficial topographic anatomy, particularly as it relates to the disposition of underlying structures, is of inestimable value to the physician and therapist. The reasons why this is so will become more apparent to you as you progress in your training. Suffice it to say that portions of many bones and muscles and even some nerves, vessels and internal organs are visible or palpable through the skin.

Although the tissues of the cadaver are less pliable than those of the living, much can be learned by careful **visual inspection** and by **palpation** of a given region before removing the skin and superficial fascia. When possible and practical, instructions for palpation of the cadaver should be performed first upon the living; that is, upon yourself and a willing colleague.

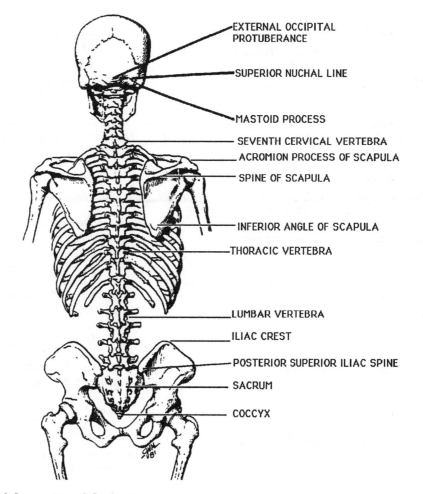

EXTERNAL OCCIPITAL PROTUBERANCE

SUPERIOR NUCHAL LINE

MASTOID PROCESS

SEVENTH CERVICAL VERTEBRA

ACROMION PROCESS OF SCAPULA

SPINE OF SCAPULA

INFERIOR ANGLE OF SCAPULA

THORACIC VERTEBRA

LUMBAR VERTEBRA

ILIAC CREST

POSTERIOR SUPERIOR ILIAC SPINE

SACRUM

COCCYX

Figure 2:1 Osteologic features of the region of the back.

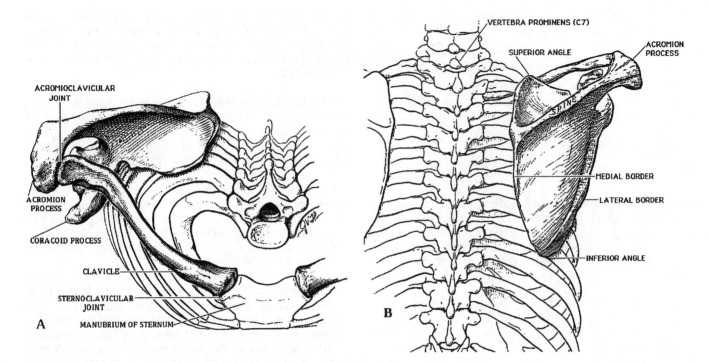

Figure 2:2 The pectoral girdle: scapula and clavicle. Selected features of the bones of the pectoral girdle and adjacent bones. A, from above; B, from behind.

Osteology. *Identify the following osseous features upon individual bones and an articulated skeleton, then palpate as many of these as you can.* The items listed can be seen in Figures 2:1, 2:2.

Skull:
    mastoid process
    external occipital protuberance
    superior nuchal line

Vertebral Column:
    spine of the vertebra prominens (the spinous process of the seventh cervical or first thoracic vertebra)
    spines of the thoracic and lumbar vertebrae
    sacrum
    coccyx

Pectoral Girdle:
    clavicle
    scapula

Clavicle:
    medial and lateral extremities
    shaft
    curvatures

Scapula:
    acromion process (the "tip" of the shoulder)
    spine of the scapula
    medial or vertebral border

    inferior angle
    lateral or axillary border
    coracoid process
    superior angle

With a pencil or sharp pointed instrument, inscribe the following lines upon the skin of the cadaver (Figure 2:3):

1. From the external occipital protuberance, down the midline of the back to the tip of the coccyx.

2. Laterally, from the external occipital protuberance to the mastoid process on each side of the cadaver.

3. Laterally, from the spine of the vertebra prominens (spine of C7 or T1) to the acromion process of each shoulder.

4. Superiorly from the coccyx, curving obliquely to the iliac crests in the midaxillary line on each side of the body; that is, to a point about halfway around the upper edge of each hipbone.

Incise the skin along the lines described above and reflect it laterally. Take precautions to avoid cutting too deeply with the scalpel; in some bodies the superficial fascia is quite thin and more deeply situated structures can be easily cut and destroyed.

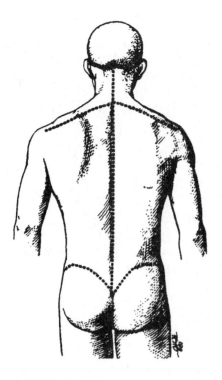

Figure 2:3 Skin incisions.

*Reflect the skin and the superficial fascia (tela subcutanea) bilaterally; that is, on both sides of the cadaver. Care must be taken to avoid going too deeply, to avoid damage to the underlying muscles (Fig. 2:4), especially the **trapezius** and **latissimus dorsi** muscles and their aponeuroses. Identify these before the skin and fascia are reflected more than a few centimeters.*

*As the superficial fascia is being reflected, watch for the emergence of **neurovascular bundles** from the deep fascia within a few centimeters from the midline, thereafter passing into the deep surface of the superficial fascia. Save short segments of several of these for later demonstration and review.*

*Remove enough deep fascia to clarify the borders of the two most superficial muscles of the extrinsic muscles of the back, the **trapezius** and the **latissimus dorsi** (Fig. 2:4).*

Components of Neurovascular Bundles. A neurovascular bundle consists of a small **artery**, a small **nerve** (here, a cutaneous nerve) and one or more small **veins** - all of which are held together by connective tissue. Only the most careful dissection, perhaps aided by a hand lens, would demonstrate these individual components clearly.

The vascular components of the neurovascular bundles consist of **cutaneous branches** of deeper arteries and **tributaries** to deeper veins. The deep arteries and veins, segmentally distributed to the body wall, are named cervical, intercostal, lumbar or

sacral arteries or veins, depending upon their location. Remember, arteries are described as having **branches** because of the direction of flow of the blood within them; veins, conversely, are said to have **tributaries.**

The neural components of the segmentally arising neurovascular bundles provide the cutaneous nerves of the posterior surface of the neck and back. These are terminal portions of the posterior (dorsal) primary rami of spinal nerves (Figures 2:5,6).

Cutaneous nerves perform two important functions:

1. They convey **sensations** (via sensory fibers from the skin – such as touch, pressure, temperature, and pain.

2. They carry **autonomic motor** nerve fibers which innervate smooth muscle in the walls of superficial blood vessels, the pilomotor muscles associated with hair rootlets, and the sweat and sebaceous glands of the skin. These autonomic fibers are postganglionic sympathetic axons which have their cell bodies in sympathetic chain ganglia.

Intrinsic and Extrinsic Muscles of the Back. A number of the muscles which you will encounter first in your dissection are included among those which are referred to as "extrinsic" muscles; that is, even though you see them on the dorsal surface of the body, their functions pertain principally to movements of the upper limbs or the ribs - not to movements of the vertebral column. Muscles seen in the back region which act primarily to flex, extend, or bend the vertebral column in lateral or oblique directions are referred to, collectively, as "intrinsic" muscles of the back.

In addition to being divided into intrinsic and extrinsic muscles, the musculature of the back can be separated by the relative depth of muscles into superficial, intermediate and deep muscle layers. The extrinsic muscles of the upper limbs and ribs comprise the superficial and intermediate layers.

Superficial Musculature. The first two muscles to be exposed are both extrinsic muscles of the back and form a superficial layer of muscle. The trapezius and the latissimus dorsi muscles are related functionally to movements of the pectoral girdle of the upper limb - **not** movements of the back. Embryologically, the superficial muscles migrate to their definitive positions, taking their nerve supply with them; thus, neither of these muscles receives supply from the dorsal primary rami in the region.

The trapezius muscle is supplied by the **spinal accessory nerve,** one of the cranial nerves. It receives supplementary nerve supply from cervical nerves C3 and C4 which is probably sensory in nature. The latissimus dorsi is supplied by the

30

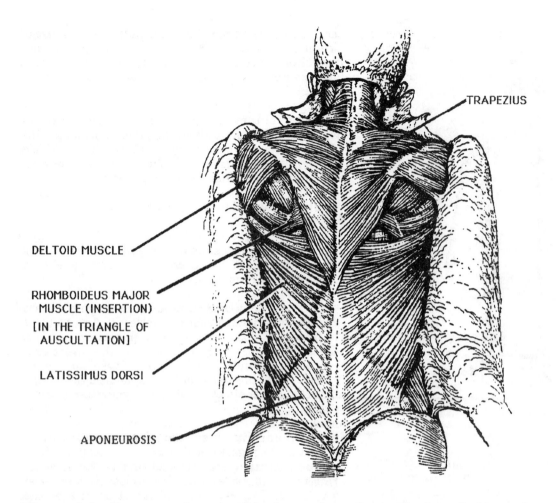

TRAPEZIUS

DELTOID MUSCLE

RHOMBOIDEUS MAJOR
MUSCLE (INSERTION)
[IN THE TRIANGLE OF
AUSCULTATION]

LATISSIMUS DORSI

APONEUROSIS

Figure 2:4 Exposure of extrinsic back muscles, after reflection of skin and superficial fascia. The rhomboideus major lies in the floor of the "triangle of auscultation" - bordered by the trapezius, latissimus dorsi and the medial border of the scapula - where a stethoscope can be applied to the chest wall to better hear the sounds of the heart and lungs.

thoracodorsal nerve, a nerve which arises from the brachial plexus of the upper limb. The spinal accessory nerve and the thoracodorsal nerve will be dissected later.

The **trapezius** muscle arises from the base of the skull, the ligamentum nuchae (a thick, ligamentous band in the midline of the neck dorsally), and spinous processes of vertebrae C7 - T12 (Table 2:1). The muscle inserts upon the lateral third of the clavicle and the acromion process and spine of the scapula. The trapezius is important in scapular movements and movements of the upper limb, such as shrugging the shoulders, rotating the shoulder upward (as when one lifts the arm above the level of the shoulders) and so on.

The **latissimus dorsi** muscle arises from spines of the lower thoracic, lumbar and sacral vertebrae, the posterior part of the iliac crest and the lower four ribs (Table 2:1). It inserts upon the intertubercular groove of the humerus - acting to extend and adduct the arm and to rotate it medially. This muscle is particularly active in exercises such as chinups.

*While cleaning away the tough fascia that overlies the most cephalic portion of the trapezius, look for and preserve the **greater occipital nerve**. This nerve can usually be found approximately one inch from the midline of the neck about one inch inferior to the superior nuchal line, as the nerve pierces the trapezius. Locate the **occipital artery** and preserve it as the trapezius is reflected. The occipital artery joins the greaater occipital nerve in this region and courses with it, supplying the scalp.*

Detach the trapezius from its origin upon the superior nuchal line and the external occipital protuberance, and sever those fibers that arise from the spines and associated ligaments of the cervical and thoracic vertebrae. Reflect the trapezius laterally toward its insertion upon the scapula.

*Make an incision through the aponeurosis of the latissimus dorsi about one-half inch from the midline of the back and also cut its attachment to the crest of the ilium. Reflect this muscle superiorly and laterally. If you do not exercise care, you will reflect the **serratus posterior inferior muscle** with the*

31

latissimus dorsi. The key to their separation lies in the recognition of the fact that although the serratus posterior inferior arises in common with part of the latissimus dorsi, the serratus posterior inferior inserts upon the lower ribs. These fibers can be observed as they diverge from those of the latissimus to pass to their insertion. Cut the origin of this serratus muscle and reflect it toward its insertion.

The Intermediate Layer of Muscles. The serratus posterior inferior is the first of the so-called intermediate layer of muscles to be exposed. The intermediate layer of muscles includes the serratus posterior inferior, levator scapulae, rhomboideus major, rhomboideus minor and the serratus posterior superior. They all receive motor nerve supply from ventral primary rami of spinal nerves. Consult Table 2:1 for the attachments (origin and insertion), function and specific nerve supply of each of these muscles. The levator scapulae and rhomboid muscles in general attach to, and move, the scapula. The serratus muscles insert upon the ribs and are of minor significance in breathing.

*Having first reflected the trapezius, identify the **levator scapulae, rhomboideus minor** and the **rhomboideus major muscles**. Cut the rhomboideus major and minor at their origins from the spines and the supraspinous ligaments of the lower cervical and upper thoracic vertebrae. Clean the fascia from these muscles so that their fibers can be seen clearly. In some specimens the line of cleavage between the two rhomboid muscles can be unclear. As necessary, consult the summary description of the muscles of the back (Table 2:1) to learn the exact attachments of these two muscles and then separate them accordingly.*

*Turn the rhomboid muscles toward their insertions upon the medial border of the scapula and, deep to them, identify the **serratus posterior superior**. Like the serratus posterior inferior, referred to above, the **serratus posterior superior** inserts upon the ribs, rather than upon the scapula. This fact should assist you in its identification. Sever the fibers of origin of this muscle and reflect it toward its insertion.*

The Greater Occipital Nerve. The greater occipital nerve is the medial branch of the dorsal primary ramus of the second cervical spinal nerve (DPR of C2). This nerve provides most of the cutaneous fibers for the posterior one-half of the scalp. Before it enters the superficial fascia and becomes a cutaneous nerve, however, the greater occipital nerve provides motor supply to the intrinsic back muscles through which it passes.

The Occipital Artery. The occipital artery arises from the external carotid artery near the angle of the mandible. After arising there, the occipital artery passes posteriorly deep to the sternocleidomastoid muscle and between deep intrinsic muscles of the neck, emerging to a subcutaneous position between the sternocleidomastoid and trapezius muscles. Thereafter, the artery travels with the greater occipital nerve and supplies tissues of the scalp posteriorly.

The Thoracolumbar Fascia. The musculature of the back is invested with, and in some areas has important attachment to layers of deep fascia. The deep fascia of the neck is called **nuchal fascia**. (The word **nuchal** refers to the neck.) Inferiorly this fascia is continuous with fascia that invests the thoracic and lumbar back musculature and is therefore called **thoracolumbar fascia**.

In the thoracic region, where the thoracolumbar fascia is relatively thin, it ensheathes the aponeurotic origin of the serratus posterior superior. In the lumbar region the thoracolumbar fascia consists of posterior, intermediate and anterior layers which enclose the intrinsic back muscles. The posterior layer is thickened considerably by its fusion with the aponeuroses of several muscles, including the latissimus dorsi.

The Intrinsic Muscles of the Back. The intrinsic muscles of the back include the splenius muscles, the erector spinae muscle group, the transversospinalis muscle group and the segmental muscles.

*On the dorsum of the neck, deep to the trapezius, identify the **splenius muscle**.* This is the first of the four major groups of intrinsic muscles in the back. The splenius consists of two parts, the **splenius cervicis** and **splenius capitis**. The two parts are named according to their insertion; that is, whether the muscle bundles insert upon the cervical vertebrae (cervicis) or upon the posterior aspect of the skull (capitis).

The splenius inclines from medial to lateral as its fibers ascend from ligamentum nuchae or vertebral spines to insertion upon the occipital bone or transverse processes of more superior vertebrae. The name splenius is based upon the resemblance of the muscle to a bandage wrapped around the neck posteriorly.

*Make a longitudinal incision through the lumbar part of the thoracolumbar fascia near the midline and then, by cutting its attachments to the underlying musculature, reflect the fascia laterally far enough to expose the **erector spinae muscle** layer – the second major muscle group. The fascia can then be cut free and discarded. This reflection of the thoracolumbar fascia will be performed in the lumbar region only, for in the thoracic region it is unnecessary because the fascia is much thinner there.*

*Identify and separate the three longitudinally oriented columns of the erector spinae muscle: the **spinalis, longissimus** and **iliocostalis**. Then, to expose the deeper musculature, remove a block of the erector spinae muscles several inches long from the* *lower thoracic and upper lumbar region and attempt to identify the **transversospinalis musculature**.* The **transversospinalis** muscles include the **semispinalis, multifidus** and **rotatores**.

The fourth general group of intrinsic muscles consists of the **segmental muscles,** including **interspinales** and **intertransversarii**. These need not be identified.

The Erector Spinae Muscle. The erector spinae muscle layer, the second major grouping of intrinsic muscles, consists of three poorly demarcated columns of muscle. From medial to lateral these are the **spinalis,** the **longissimus** and the **iliocostalis**.

The **spinalis muscle** can be identified by the fact that its individual muscle bundles arise from, and insert upon vertebral spines. It is best seen in the mid-thoracic region. Even there, its more lateral fibers blend with the adjacent longissimus muscle.

The **longissimus** is the intermediate part of the erector spinae group and is the largest and longest segment of the intrinsic musculature; it can be seen to extend from the lumbar region to the base of the skull. Its fibers blend medially with the spinalis in the thoracic region; they intermingle laterally with the various parts of the iliocostalis muscle in the lumbar, thoracic and cervical regions.

The longissimus is divided into thoracic, cervical and head (capitis) segments. Longissimus thoracis arises from the common tendon of the erector spinae and inserts into the lower nine or ten ribs and adjacent transverse processes. Longissimus cervicis arises from the upper four to six thoracic vertebrae and inserts into the transverse processes of cervical vertebrae 2-6. Longissimus capitis arises from the insertion of cervicis and inserts into the mastoid process.

The iliocostalis is the most lateral of the erector spinae group and is subdivided into three linear but overlapping segments; lumborum arises mainly from the iliac crest and sacrum and inserts into the lower six or seven ribs. The iliocostalis thoracis arises from these same ribs and inserts into the upper six ribs. The iliocostalis cervicis arises from these ribs and inserts into the transverse processes of the fourth to sixth cervical vertebrae.

The Transversospinalis Muscle Group. The third group of intrinsic muscles, the transversospinalis musculature, includes **semispinalis, multifidus** and **rotator muscles**. Longitudinally, these fill in the concavity between the tips of the transverse processes and the spinous processes of the vertebrae. In general, their individual muscle bundles incline medially and superiorly from their origins to their insertions.

The **semispinalis muscle** includes the **semispinalis thoracis, cervicis** and **capitis** - each part named according to its location. Semispinalis muscle bundles typically arise from the transverse process of one vertebra and ascend about six vertebral levels to insert upon a spinous process. In the dorsum of the neck, the semispinalis capitis forms a thick, vertically oriented layer of muscle lying just deep to the splenius muscle.

The **multifidus muscle** lies deep to the erector spinae and to the semispinalis, where its fibers arise from transverse processes and adjacent parts of the vertebrae. Bundles of this muscle ascend about three to five vertebral levels before inserting upon spinous processes of higher vertebrae. The deeper fascicles of this muscle are successively shorter, becoming indistinguishable from the deeper members of the transversospinalis, the **rotatores**. The **long** and **short rotator muscles** ascend two or one vertebral levels, respectively, between origin and insertion. The rotator muscles are seen best in the thoracic region.

Actions of the Intrinsic Muscles. The function of the intrinsic muscles can be summarized as follows:

Splenius - Turns face to the same side as the contracting muscle. Bilateral contraction results in extension of the neck.

Erector spinae - Unilateral contraction causes lateral flexion of vertebral column to same side with some rotation to that side; bilateral contraction produces extension of column.

Transversospinalis - Contraction bilaterally causes extension; unilateral contraction produces rotation to the opposite side. The semispinalis capitis can turn the head toward the opposite side.

Nerve Supply of Intrinsic Back Muscles. All intrinsic back muscles receive their motor and sensory innervation by way of **dorsal primary rami** of the spinal nerves.

Spinal Nerves

In preceding descriptions of the motor and sensory innervation of structures in the back, mention was made of dorsal and ventral primary rami and their relative contributions to the sensory and motor innervation of the structures of the back. The rami referred to are the principal branches of the nerves which arise from the spinal cord – the **spinal nerves**. We will now examine the functional anatomy of spinal nerves in somewhat greater detail. Understanding of much to come depends upon a working knowledge of these facts.

Thirty-one pairs of spinal nerves arise segmentally from the spinal cord – including eight cervical, twelve thoracic, five lumbar, five sacral and one coccygeal pair. Each pair of spinal nerves arises from a **segment** or **neuromere** of the spinal cord by a

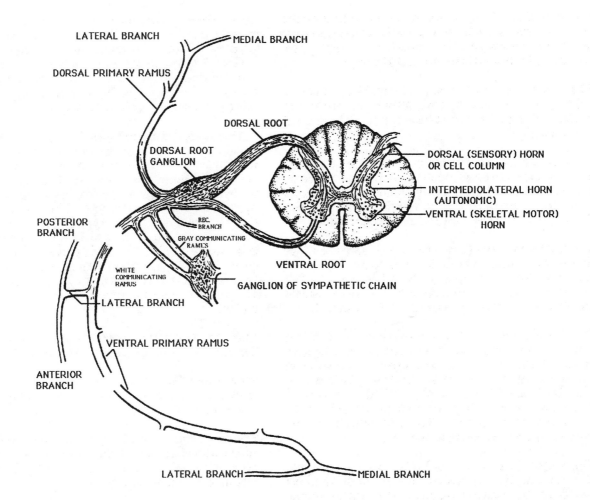

LATERAL BRANCH — MEDIAL BRANCH
DORSAL PRIMARY RAMUS
DORSAL ROOT
DORSAL ROOT GANGLION
DORSAL (SENSORY) HORN OR CELL COLUMN
INTERMEDIOLATERAL HORN (AUTONOMIC)
VENTRAL (SKELETAL MOTOR) HORN
POSTERIOR BRANCH
REC. BRANCH
GRAY COMMUNICATING RAMUS
WHITE COMMUNICATING RAMUS
VENTRAL ROOT
LATERAL BRANCH
GANGLION OF SYMPATHETIC CHAIN
VENTRAL PRIMARY RAMUS
ANTERIOR BRANCH
LATERAL BRANCH — MEDIAL BRANCH

Figure 2:5 Schematic drawing of a typical spinal nerve. The ventral root contains skeletal motor and autonomic fibers (the latter only in spinal nerves T1 - L2 and S2 - S4.). The dorsal root contains only sensory fibers. The dorsal and ventral primary rami are "mixed" nerves, containing all three types of fibers.

number of rootlets. The first cervical spinal nerve emerges from the spinal canal between the atlas (the first vertebra) and the base of the skull. The other spinal nerves are formed at the intervertebral foramen present between each two adjacent vertebrae.

There are obvious differences between various spinal nerves, such as their specific types of fiber composition, external appearance, and branching patterns. Nevertheless, sufficient similarities exist among spinal nerves in general that one can describe what is called a "typical" spinal nerve.

A **typical spinal nerve** is formed by the union of **ventral** and **dorsal roots** which are attached to the spinal cord (Fig. 2:5) by rootlets, as noted above. The **ventral root** carries motor fibers; in fact, every ventral root contains skeletal motor axons, the cell bodies of which are located in a spinal cord nucleus called the **ventral motor horn**. The axons are carried by the ventral root to the spinal nerve trunk, after which they can enter either the ventral primary

ramus or the dorsal primary ramus for distribution to skeletal muscles.

In addition to somatic motor fibers, the ventral root of certain spinal nerves contains preganglionic autonomic axons. These spinal nerves include levels T1 – L2 with their sympathetic neurons and S2 – S4, with their parasympathetic neurons. The cell bodies of these autonomic neurons are located in a nucleus located at these levels called the **intermediolateral cell column (IML).**

The **dorsal root** of the spinal nerve carries sensory fibers, and characteristically possesses a slight swelling, the **dorsal root ganglion**. This ganglion contains the **pseudounipolar cell bodies** of the sensory fibers. Each cell body possesses a **peripheral** process and a **central** process. That part of the dorsal root between the ganglion and the spinal cord consists of the central processes of the sensory cell bodies in the ganglion. The peripheral processes of these neurons pass out into the branches (dorsal and ventral rami) of the spinal nerve. The peripheral process carries sensory information from

34

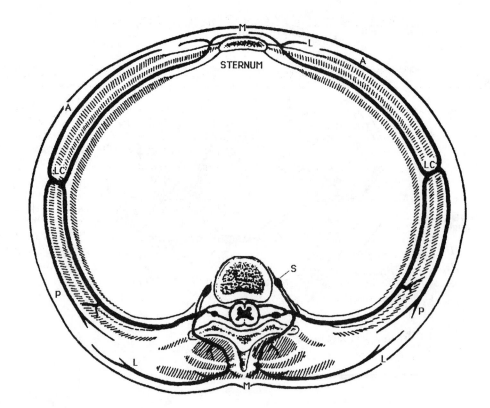

Figure 2:6 Schematic drawing of the relationships of a "typical spinal nerve" to the body wall. LC, lateral cutaneous branch of ventral primary ramus; A, anterior; P, posterior; M, medial, and L, lateral terminal cutaneous branches of rami; S, paravertebral ganglion of sympathetic chain.

the body wall, limbs or organs into the dorsal root ganglion to the cell body of the neuron; the central process then conveys this information on into the spinal cord, wherein the process may make numerous synaptic connections.

The part of the nerve representing the fusion of the dorsal and ventral root is called the **mixed spinal nerve** (or the spinal nerve **trunk**). The mixed spinal nerve is typically very short, for it divides just outside the vertebral column into a ventral primary ramus and a dorsal primary ramus. **The dorsal primary rami and ventral primary rami are all mixed nerves**; that is, all and each carry sensory, skeletal motor, and autonomic fibers.

The **dorsal** (or, posterior) **primary rami** of the spinal nerves supply the intrinsic back musculature and the skin of the back. The **ventral** (anterior) **primary rami** of the spinal nerves supply the skin and musculature of the remainder of the body wall and, furthermore, through the formation of various plexuses (cervical, brachial, lumbar, sacral and coccygeal), supply sensory and motor innervation to the upper and lower limbs.

The **ventral primary rami** of spinal nerves are connected to the sympathetic ganglionated chains by means of small nerve branches called **communicating rami.** It is by means of such connections between vertebral levels T1 and L2 that all sympathetic preganglionic fibers get from the spinal cord to the sympathetic chains for synapse there or elsewhere. Communicating rami also carry postganglionic sympathetic fibers from the ganglia of the chain to every one of the spinal nerves for distribution to the blood vessels, pilomotor muscles and glands of the skin in the body wall and limbs.

In actuality, only a few spinal nerves exhibit all of the characteristics illustrated of the "typical" spinal nerve shown in Figures 2:5 and 2:6. For instance, the dorsal primary ramus of C1 has no cutaneous distribution, and the ventral primary rami of C5-T1 have essentially no distribution to the skin of the neck or thorax, being incorporated into the brachial plexus for supply of the upper limb.

TABLE 2:1 The Extrinsic Muscles of the Back.

MUSCLES	ATTACHMENTS	FUNCTIONS	INNERVATION
Trapezius	Origin: superior nuchal line; ligamentum nuchae and spines of C7–T12 Insertion: lateral portion of clavicle; spine of the scapula	Elevation, depression, upward (medial) and downward (lateral) rotation, retraction (adduction) of the scapula. By elevating the glenoid cavity, it aids in elevating arm.	Spinal accessory nerve (CN XI), C3, C4 (VPR) (ventral primary rami)
Latissimus dorsi	Origin: spines of T6–sacral vertebrae, inclusive; posterior portion of iliac crest; lower four ribs Insertion: intertubercular groove of humerus; inferior angle of scapula	Extension, medial rotation and adduction of arm.	Thoracodorsal nerve (a branch of the brachial plexus)
Levator scapulae	Origin: transverse processes of C1-C4 Insertion: medial border and superior angle of the scapula	Elevation and lateral (downward) rotation of scapula	Dorsal scapular nerve (a branch of the brachial plexus); C3 and C4
Rhomboideus minor	Origin: ligamentum nuchae and spines of C7, T1 Insertion: medial border of scapula at, and above, the root of spine of scapula	Retraction (adduction) and elevation of the scapula	Dorsal scapular nerve (a branch of the brachial plexus)
Rhomboideus major	Origin: spines of T2–T5 Insertion: medial border of scapula below its spine.	Retraction (adduction) and elevation of the scapula	Dorsal scapular nerve (a branch of the brachial plexus)
Serratus posterior superior	Origin; spines of C7-T3 and the supraspinous ligament Insertion: ribs 2–5	Elevation of ribs 2 - 5	Intercostal nerves (ventral primary rami)
Serratus posterior inferior	Origin: spines of T11-L3 and the supraspinous ligament Insertion: ribs 9-12	Depression of ribs 9 - 12	Intercostal nerves (VPR)

TABLE 2:2 The Intrinsic Muscles of the Back.

MUSCLES	ATTACHMENTS	FUNCTIONS	INNERVATION
Splenius- capitis, cervicis	Origin: ligamentum nuchae; spines C7–T6 Insertion: skull, upper cervical transverse processes.	Turns head to same side; extends neck	Local dorsal primary rami (DPR)
Erector Spinae: Iliocostalis— lumborum thoracis, cervicis, capitis Longissimus— thoracis, cervicis, capitis Spinalis - thoracis, cervicis, capitis	Origin: vertebral spines; sacrum, ilium and ribs – variable, depending upon specific muscle component involved. Insertion: skull, ribs, spines and transverse processes of vertebrae	Extend vertebral column, selectively flexes column laterally.	Local dorsal primary rami (DPR)
Transversospinalis: Semispinalis— thoracis, cervicis, capitis	Origin: Transverse processes, variably, depending upon the specific muscle component involved. Semispinalis capitis inserts on the occipital bone of the skull.	Semispinalis capitis rotates the head to the opposite side. Other transversospinalis muscles extend vertebral column and rotate column.	Local dorsal primary rami (DPR)
Multifidus sacral, lumbar, thoracic, cervical Rotatores— longi, breves	Insertions: Spinous processes of higher vertebrae. Semispinalis inserts six or more levels higher; multifidus 3 - 5 levels higher; long rotators 2 above; short rotators, next higher spinous process		

Questions for review and study

1. What two types of nerve fibers are carried by cutaneous nerves?

Sensory and autonomic (sympathetic postganglionic) fibers.

2. What functions are performed by the autonomic fibers in cutaneous nerves?

They provide motor supply to the smooth muscle of blood vessels, pilomotor muscles and sweat glands.

3. The cutaneous veins are branches of deeper veins. True or false?

False. They are **tributaries** to deeper veins.

4. What bones form the pectoral girdle?

The two scapulae and the two clavicles.

5. What is the upper, or superior limb?

Arm, forearm and hand - also termed the brachium, antebrachium and hand

6. What is the origin of the greater occipital nerve?

The dorsal primary ramus of C2. Its medial branch, in particular, is known as the greater occipital nerve.

7. What is the distribution of the dorsal primary ramus of the first cervical nerve?

The dorsal primary ramus of C1 supplies muscles in the immediate area; it has no cutaneous distribution. Its dorsal root ganglion is therefore very small.

8. What is the origin of the occipital artery?

The occipital artery arises from the external carotid artery.

9. What are the region of distribution and the functions of the greater occipital nerve?

The greater occipital nerve is a cutaneous nerve for the posterior portion of the scalp. It also supplies intrinsic back muscles before it enters the superficial fascia.

10. What types of nerve fibers are contained within a typical dorsal primary ramus?

A DPR contains sensory, postganglionic sympathetic and skeletal motor fibers. After distribution of its skeletal motor fibers the DPR continues as a cutaneous nerve.

11. What types of nerve fibers are contained within a typical ventral primary ramus?

A VPR contains the same types of fibers as a DPR, except that certain VPR also contain preganglionic autonomic fibers. [Sympathetic: T1-L2; Parasympathetic: S2-S4]

12. What is a mixed nerve?

A mixed nerve contains more than one functional type of nerve fiber. Most named nerves are mixed nerves. All DPR and VPR are mixed nerves, too.

13. From what bones does the trapezius arise?

The posterior part of the skull; spines of cervical and thoracic vertebrae.

14. Upon what bony features does the trapezius insert?

The lateral third of the clavicle and the acromion process and spine of the scapula

15. What is the one major difference between ligaments and tendons?

Ligaments join bones to bones; tendons join muscles to bones.

16. What is the ligamentum nuchae?

The ligamentum nuchae is a portion of the supraspinous ligament - which is especially thick in the nuchal region (nape), or posterior part of the neck.

17. What bones form the pelvic girdle?

The innominate (hip) bones, joined at the pubic symphysis, form the pelvic girdle. Each hip bone is composed of three fused bones - the pubic bone, ischium and ilium.

18. What is an aponeurosis? Give examples.

Aponeuroses are flattened tendons. Both the trapezius and latissimus dorsi take origin in part by aponeurotic tendons which attach to vertebral spinous processes.

19. What are the three divisions of the erector spinae muscle?

The spinalis, longissimus, iliocostalis

20. What is the innervation of all intrinsic back muscles?

Skeletal motor branches of dorsal primary rami.

21. What is the insertion of the latissimus dorsi?

The humerus - the bone of the brachium. It also has a small attachment to the inferior angle of the scapula.

22. Upon what bones do the serratus posterior superior and inferior insert?

They insert upon ribs

23. What layer of fascia is associated with the intrinsic muscles of the back in the thoracic and lumbar areas?

The thoracolumbar fascia

24. Where are the cell bodies of sensory fibers which supply the skin of the back?

The cell bodies of sensory fibers from the back are located in dorsal root ganglia.

25. Where are the cell bodies of the motor axons which supply the erector spinae muscle?

The cell bodies of the motor fibers for the erector spinae muscle are located in the ventral cell column of the spinal cord.

26. What types of nerve fibers are found in dorsal roots of spinal nerves?

Sensory fibers only.

27. What types of nerve fibers are found in ventral roots of spinal nerves?

Skeletal motor fibers and, at certain spinal levels, autonomic fibers. Ventral roots at levels T1-L2 contain preganglionic sympathetic axons; ventral roots at S2-S4 contain preganglionic parasympathetic axons.

28. Upon what bone do the levator scapulae, rhomboideus minor and rhomboideus major insert?

The scapula, on its medial aspect (vertebral border). The levator scapulae inserts upon the superior angle of the scapula.

29. What is the origin of a muscle?

The bony attachment of a muscle which remains relatively immobile when the muscle contracts is referred to as its origin.

30 What is the insertion of a muscle?

The bony attachment of a muscle which undergoes some degree of movement when the muscle contracts is known as its insertion.

LABORATORY IDENTIFICATION CHECK-LIST

Superficial Dissection of the Back

The following list contains the names of structures which you are expected to find on the cadaver, or other laboratory materials. You may notice additional structures named in the text which are not included here; you can assume these to be of lesser importance, or as items which require too much time for identification with certainty.

skull
mastoid process
external occipital protuberance
superior nuchal line

vertebral column
vertebra prominens - spine of C7 or T1
spines of cervical, thoracic, lumbar vertebrae
sacrum
coccyx

scapula
acromion process
spine of scapula
vertebral border of scapula
axillary border of scapula
superior angle
inferior angle
coracoid process

clavicle
sternal end
acromial end
curvatures

innominate bone
crest of ilium

superficial fascia
deep fascia
neurovascular bundles

trapezius
latissimus dorsi

greater occipital nerve
occipital artery
serratus posterior inferior
levator scapulae
rhomboideus minor
rhomboideus major
serratus posterior superior
thoracolumbar fascia

splenius

erector spinae
spinalis
longissimus
iliocostalis

transversospinalis
  semispinalis
  multifidus
  rotatores

Coccyx [Gr. *kokkyx* , cuckoo, whose bill this bone is said to resemble]
The small bone caudad to the sacrum in man, formed by the union of four (sometimes five or three) rudimentary vertebrae, and forming the caudal extremity of the vertebral column.

Latissimus [L. *latus,* broad]
A general term denoting a broad structure muscle such as the latissimus dorsi muscle.

Neurovascular - Pertaining to both neural (nerve) and vascular elements.

Prominens - A protrusion or projection.

Ramus (pl. rami) [L. a branch]
A general term for a smaller structure given off by a larger one, or into which the larger structure, such as a blood vessel or nerve, divides.

CHAPTER 3

THE SPINAL CORD AND THE SUBOCCIPITAL TRIANGLE

In this dissection much of the intrinsic musculature of the back and portions of the vertebrae will be removed to expose the meninges (membranous coverings of the CNS), the spinal cord and spinal nerves. Before attempting the dissection, study the details of the architecture of the vertebrae (Figures 3:1-6).

Osteology. The vertebral column, or backbone, consists of the **seven cervical vertebrae, twelve thoracic vertebrae, five lumbar vertebrae,** the **sacrum** (which represents the five fused **sacral vertebrae**) and the **coccyx** (composed of three to five fused vertebrae).

The vertebral column in the fetus is C-shaped (when viewed from the right side), flexed in a ventral direction. This curvature is called the **primary curvature** of the spine. Its shape is retained in the adult in the thoracic and sacro-coccygeal areas of the vertebral column. After birth, **secondary curvatures** develop; first, in the cervical region when the baby begins lifting its head; second, in the lumbar region with the assumption of upright posture and walking.

Increases in the convexity of the primary curvature of the thoracic spine from disease or ageing produce **kyphosis** (hunchback). Increases in the secondary curvatures, particularly in the lumbar region - are referred to as **lordosis** and as lordotic curves. The vertebral column can also exhibit lateral curvatures; these are referred to as **scoliosis**, and are observed most commonly in adolescent girls. A slight degree of scoliotic curvature is not abnormal, is often associated with right - or left handedness, and goes usually undetected.

A typical vertebra consists of a **body** and a **vertebral arch** which, together, enclose an opening, the **vertebral foramen.** The collective vertebral foramina of the vertebral column form the **vertebral canal** (or, **spinal canal**), in which the spinal cord and its coverings lie.

Subjacent vertebrae are held apart and joined together by the **intervertebral disks** (Fig. 3:9). The combined thicknesses of these account for about one-quarter of the total length of the vertebral column. An intervertebral disk consists of an outer **anulus fibrosis**, composed of dense connective tissue and fibrocartilage, and a central portion, the **nucleus pulposus**, consisting of a soft, gelatinous substance. It is presumed that the nucleus pulposus is retained from the embryologic **notochord**.

With degeneration or shearing of the anulus fibrosus, and under compressive forces, the nucleus pulposus can be forced through fissures in the anulus - extruding through it much as toothpaste from a tube, although firmer in consistency. Thereafter, the extruded nucleus pulposus can press against spinal nerves or their parts, or even against the spinal cord in some cases (a more serious problem, clinically). This eruption of the nucleus pulposus from the intervertebral disk is known as **disk herniation** or, more colloquially, **ruptured disk**.

Typical Vertebra. The most common type of vertebra is one which possesses two main bony parts (Fig. 3:1-5):

1. The **vertebral body** - generally, the most massive part of the vertebra, and rather cylindrical in form. Vertebral bodies are the weight bearing portions of the vertebrae; adjacent vertebral bodies are separated from one another by the intervertebral disks.

2. The **vertebral arch** (or, **neural arch**) - forms the sides and roof of the vertebral canal, with the vertebral body forming a floor for the canal. The sides of the vertebral arch consist of two **pedicles**, each pedicle possessing a **superior vertebral notch** and an **inferior notch**. The inferior vertebral notch of one vertebra and the superior vertebral notch of an adjacent vertebra in large measure form the boundaries of an **intervertebral foramen.** The spinal nerves leave the spinal canal by passing through the intervertebral foramina.

The **roof** of the vertebral arch is formed by a pair of **laminae** which are fused in the midline.

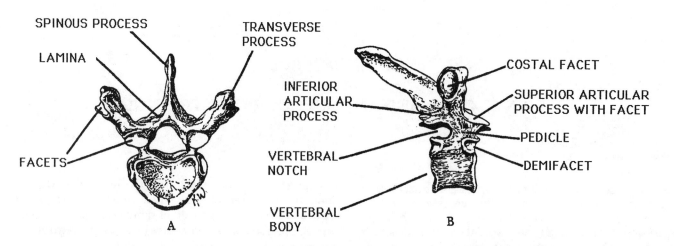

Figure 3:1 A typical thoracic vertebra. A, view from above; B, viewed from the right side.

The vertebral arch provides origin for three types of processes: the **spinous process**, two **transverse processes**, and two pairs of **articular processes** (or, **zygopophyses**). The spinous process projects posteriorly from the junction of the two laminae and provides a site of attachment for muscles and vertebral ligaments. The transverse process projects laterally from the junction of the lamina and pedicle of each side of the vertebra; these also figure prominently in the attachments of intrinsic muscles and, in the thoracic region, provide sites of articulation for ribs.

The majority of vertebrae possess **superior** and **inferior articular processes** for the articulation of adjacent vertebrae. The superior articular processes face posteriorly and the inferior processes are directed anteriorly, although the exact orientation of the processes varies from one region of the vertebral column to another. At sites of **zygopophyseal joints** the articulating surfaces, or **facets**, of the articular processes are covered with **hyaline cartilage**. These joints limit and determine the directions of movement allowed between different vertebrae. They are typical **synovial joints** of the **plane** or **gliding** variety; that is, they permit simple sliding movements of the bony surfaces against one another.

The characteristics of vertebrae from each region of the vertebral column will now be considered. Because most of them fit the picture of the "typical" vertebra well, the thoracic vertebrae will be inspected first.

Observations of vertebral features: Thoracic vertebrae. *Upon a vertebra from the midthoracic portion of the vertebral column, identify the* **spinous process**, *the* **transverse processes** *and the* **laminae** *which connect these (Fig. 3:1). Note the* **pedicles**, *by which the laminae are joined to the body of the vertebra. The pedicles and laminae form the vertebral arch. In the regions of junction of the lamina and the pedicles, identify the* **superior** *and* **inferior articular processes**, *with their cartilage-covered* **facets**. *Note that the pedicles possess* **superior** *and* **inferior vertebral notches**. *Identify the* **costal facet** *near the tip of each transverse process of the thoracic vertebrae and the* **demi-facets** *on the vertebral body. These facets, covered with hyaline cartilage, provide the sites of articulation of the ribs with these vertebrae.*

Cervical Vertebrae. *Upon a typical cervical vertebra, such as CV3 - CV6 (third to sixth cervical vertebrae), identify the* **foramen transversarium** *in each transverse process. The vertebral arteries - important arteries in the blood supply of the brain - ascend in the neck bilaterally through these foramina. Identify the* **vertebral spine** *and note that this process tends to be irregularly bifid (doubled) at its tip in the cervical region (Fig. 3:2).*

Identify the **atlas**, *the first cervical vertebra (Fig. 3:3). This vertebra gets its name from the fact that it bears the weight of the head, as the mythologic Atlas bore the weight of the earth. Note that the atlas does not have a body, nor a spine; instead, it possesses*

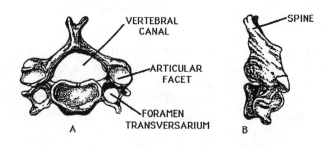

Figure 3:2 Cervical vertebra. A, viewed from above; B, viewed from the right side.

45

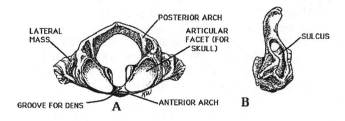

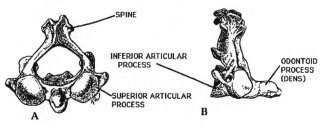

Figure 3:3 The atlas. A, superior view; B, right lateral view. The articular facets shown in A articulate with with the occipital condyles of the skull.

Figure 3:4 The axis. A, Superior view; B, right lateral view.

anterior and posterior arches and lateral masses. Note the smooth groove upon the internal surface of the anterior arch for articulation with the odontoid process of the second cervical vertebra.

The cranial border of the posterior arch has a sulcus or groove in it, bilaterally, in which the left or right vertebral arteries lies after passing through the foramen transversarium of the transverse process of its side. After passing through this sulcus, each vertebral artery ascends through the foramen magnum to enter the cranial cavity.

*Identify the **axis**, the second cervical vertebra (Fig.3:4).* The axis is characterized by a large **spine** and by the **odontoid process** or **dens**, a very important bony process which articulates with the atlas.

Fractures of the odontoid process are not uncommon in trauma. Unless the associated trauma is severe, the patient usually survives. In a "hangman's fracture," the pedicles of the axis are broken bilaterally so that the body of the axis and the posterior elements become separated.

Examine the seventh cervical vertebra. This vertebra, closely resembling a typical thoracic, vertebra, in many cases bears the long spinous process which forms the palpable landmark, the **vertebra prominens.** Its transverse processes may be notched, rather than having complete foramina.

The vertebral arteries pass through the foramina transversaria of the first six cervical vertebrae, but not the seventh.

Clinical problems in the cervical region are not uncommon - as the number of lawsuits from "whiplash" injuries from automobile wrecks will attest. The cervical part of the spinal canal is narrow, relative to the width of the cervical spinal cord; hence, there is little excess space within the canal and spinal cord compression occurs readily.

Transection or severe compression damage to the spinal cord above C3 leads to death unless the patient is permanently ventilated, because of paralysis of the diaphragm (innervated by the phrenic nerve: C3, C4, C5). Lesions at C4 and C5 can also threaten respiratory processes in the presence of relatively mild pulmonary disease.

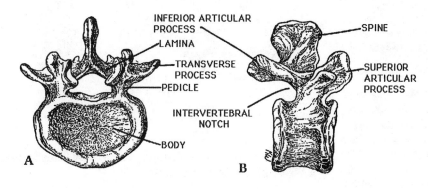

Figure 3:5 A lumbar vertebra. A, Superior view; B, right lateral view.

Vertebral degeneration and bony overgrowths can lead to irritation or compression of the cord or spinal nerve roots in the neck. Herniation of cervical intervertebral disks typically involve spinal nerves C6, C7 or C5 (in that order of frequency) with resultant clinical problems in the upper limbs.

Lumbar Vertebrae. *Note the features of lumbar vertebrae (Fig.3:5).* The typical lumbar vertebra does not possess the foramina transversaria of cervical vertebrae, nor the costal facets of thoracic vertebrae. It is quite obvious that lumbar vertebrae are more massive than either of the foregoing types, with very stout processes for the attachments of the strong, heavy musculature of the lumbar region. The fifth lumbar vertebra is in some cases fused with the sacrum, a condition referred to as **sacralization** of that vertebra.

In some individuals the fifth lumbar vertebra is separated into an anterior segment and a posterior segment, instead of being a singular, stout bone. This condition is called **spondylolysis**.

Because of the lordotic curvature of the lumbar spine, the weight of the torso in upright posture is directed vertically in front of the articulation of the fifth lumbar vertebra with the sacrum. The anterior part of the vertebra, consisting of the body and the pedicles, may break free and slide forward in front of the lumbosacral articulation, leaving the laminae, spine and inferior articular processes behind - a clinical condition known as **spondylolisthesis** (Greek, *spondylos,* vertebra + *olistheses,* a slipping and falling). The distance of slipping forward of the vertebral body is limited by ligamentous attachments; the displacement therefore results usually in pain from compression of spinal nerve roots, without narrowing of the spinal canal. The fourth lumbar vertebra can also be subject to spondylolisthesis.

Sacrum. *Upon a sacrum identify the **articular processes** for the fifth lumbar vertebra. Note the **spinous processes** and the **sacral hiatus**. Observe the forwardly concave shape (a primary curve) of the sacrum which, with the coccyx, forms the posterior bony wall of the pelvis. Note the **sacral cornua**.* The ventral portion of the body of the first sacral vertebra projects into the pelvis as the **promontory** of the sacrum. In some people the first sacral vertebra is partially or wholly separate from the remaining part of the sacrum, a condition known as **lumbarization** of S1.

*Upon the ventral surface of the sacrum identify the **ventral sacral foramina**, through which the ventral primary rami of sacral spinal nerves pass. Upon the dorsal surface, note **dorsal sacral foramina**, providing exits for the dorsal primary rami of the sacral spinal nerves.*

*On the superior lateral aspects of the sacrum identify the smooth **auricular surfaces** for*

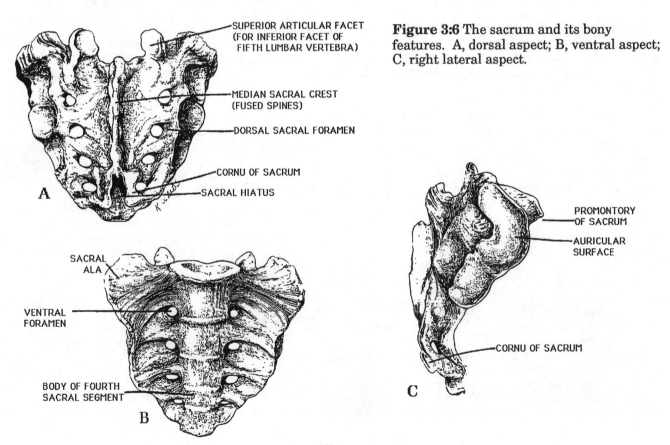

Figure 3:6 The sacrum and its bony features. A, dorsal aspect; B, ventral aspect; C, right lateral aspect.

SUPERIOR ARTICULAR FACET (FOR INFERIOR FACET OF FIFTH LUMBAR VERTEBRA)

MEDIAN SACRAL CREST (FUSED SPINES)

DORSAL SACRAL FORAMEN

CORNU OF SACRUM

SACRAL HIATUS

A

SACRAL ALA

VENTRAL FORAMEN

BODY OF FOURTH SACRAL SEGMENT

B

PROMONTORY OF SACRUM

AURICULAR SURFACE

CORNU OF SACRUM

C

articulation with the hipbones (the sacroiliac articulations). These are called auricular because they have a somewhat ear-shaped configuration. *Identify the sacral alae, large triangular areas on either side of the body of the sacrum.*

Other developmental and clinical problems: Spina Bifida. The vertebral arches and spines of vertebrae may fail to form and fuse properly in development, especially in the lower thoracic, lumbar and sacral regions. This condition, which can affect one or more vertebrae in an individual, is called **spina bifida.** This defect is often symptomless.

Spina bifida can be present with no external sign, save for the existence of a tuft of hair over the lower lumbar region - a situation known as **spina bifida occulta.** In some cases, however, the coverings of the spinal cord (the meninges) may project through such a vertebral defect, a condition referred to as **meningocele** (resembling a cyst).

If the passage of the meninges through the bony defect is accompanied by the spinal cord or nerve roots, the herniating mass is called a **meningomyelocele.** Meningoceles and meningomyeloceles must be treated surgically. **Rachischisis** is a condition in which several or all vertebrae lack closure of the vertebral arches.

Fates of Vertebral Costal Elements and Accessory Ribs. Costal (rib) elements develop in association with each vertebra, embryologically. In the thoracic region the costal elements develop into ribs. The costal elements of the seventh cervical vertebra in some individuals develop unilaterally or bilaterally into a "**cervical rib.**" Although they may be of no significance clinically, in some cases cervical ribs and/or associated connective tissue bands or accessory muscle can contribute to the development of certain neurovascular problems of the upper limb - as in, for example, the so-called **thoracic outlet syndrome** - by compression of large nerves and vessels at the root of the neck.

The costal element associated with the first lumbar vertebra in some persons can lead to the formation of an accessory rib, resulting in the presence of thirteen thoracic vertebra and only four lumbar vertebrae. Conversely, in some cases there may be only eleven thoracic vertebrae, but six lumbar vertebrae, when the costal elements of the twelfth thoracic vertebra fail to develop properly.

The costal elements of vertebrae other than the thoracic vertebrae are typically absorbed into the developing vertebral arches - forming the ventral parts of the foramina transversaria of cervical vertebrae, much of the transverse process of each lumbar vertebra and the lateral mass of the sacrum (the part lateral to the foramina, bilaterally).

The Suboccipital Region. The suboccipital region includes the structures dorsally at the base of the skull, including the elements involved in the **atlantoccipital** and **atlantoaxial** articulations, the muscles associated with the **suboccipital triangle**, the vertebral artery and veins and the first couple of cervical dorsal primary rami. The joints between the atlas and the occipital bone of the skull are associated especially with flexion and extension of the head upon the vertebral column; the atlantoaxial joints are of particular significance in rotation of the head - turning it from side to side.

Dissection. *Again identify the greater occipital nerve, the medial branch of the dorsal primary ramus of C2. After turning the trapezius away from its cephalic and cervical attachments, again note the splenius and divide it bilaterally at its origin from the spines of the cervical and upper thoracic vertebrae and reflect it laterally, exposing the semispinalis muscle. Cut the attachment of the semispinalis capitis from the skull and the ligamentum nuchae to reveal the suboccipital triangle. Preserve the greater occipital nerve as the semispinalis is reflected. Trace the nerve down through the underlying fat and tough connective tissue, clearing away the connective tissue as you do so.*

Even after the semispinalis capitis is reflected, little of the boundaries or contents of the suboccipital triangle will be immediately apparent, being hidden by overlying connective tissue and elements of a complicated plexus of veins. Remove these tissues and vessels with care, searching carefully for the small muscles which bound the triangle and taking pains to preserve them. As you follow the greater occipital nerve deeply, it will lead you to the lower border of the suboccipital triangle (to be exposed in the next part of the dissection), for it passes around the lower border of one of the muscles which bound the triangle, the inferior oblique muscle.

Identify the muscles which form the three sides of the suboccipital triangle: the inferior oblique, superior oblique and the rectus capitis posterior major. After you have identified and cleaned the rectus capitis posterior major, sever its attachment to the skull and reflect it inferiorly toward its origin from the axis to expose the rectus capitis posterior minor. This latter muscle lies deep to, and slightly medial to the former muscle. The rectus capitis posterior minor is considered to be a suboccipital muscle, but it does not contribute to the margins of the suboccipital triangle.

Within the suboccipital triangle look for branches of the suboccipital nerve, the dorsal primary ramus of C1. Clean one or more of these branches back to their origin to locate the dorsal primary ramus. This nerve emerges from the spinal canal by exiting through the interval between the base of the skull and the atlas.

When the suboccipital nerve is traced carefully, it will be seen to enter the suboccipital triangle by appearing between the vertebral artery and the posterior arch of the atlas. The C1 spinal nerve has no cutaneous distribution and is composed primarily of skeletal motor neuronal processes for supply of the suboccipital muscles and the cranial part of the semispinalis capitis.

*Locate the **posterior arch** of the **atlas** by palpation. Note the sheet of tough connective tissue which joins the posterior arch to the skull, the **posterior atlanto-occipital membrane**. Clean the loose connective tissues away from the arch to expose the **vertebral artery**, which lies in the **sulcus** of the posterior arch. This is perhaps the most important task of this part of the dissection. In order to expose and clearly demonstrate the artery, it is ordinarily necessary to remove a surrounding plexus of veins and small, anastomosing arterial branches.*

Suboccipital Vessels. After arising from the subclavian artery at the root of the neck, each **vertebral artery** enters a foramen transversarium of C6 and ascends through the foramina of the succeeding cervical vertebrae until it passes through the foramen transversarium of the atlas. It then passes through an opening in the posterior atlanto-occipital membrane and enters the skull by way of the foramen magnum. The two vertebral arteries join within the skull to form the basilar artery.

In its ascent through the neck, the vertebral artery provides small branches to the spinal cord, the spinal meninges, vertebrae and to the deep muscles. It has numerous anastomoses with other regional arteries, including the **occipital artery** and the **profunda cervicis.**

As stated previously, the **occipital artery** is a branch of the external carotid artery. Its course and distribution have also been described. The **profunda cervicis** arises from the costocervical trunk - a branch of the subclavian artery - at the root of the neck. The profunda cervicis ascends in the neck, dorsal to the transverse processes, deep to the semispinalis cervicis and capitis. In its course, it anastomoses with branches of the vertebral artery and the occipital artery.

The **vertebral vein** does not accompany the vertebral artery into the skull. Instead, the vein begins in the suboccipital region by the coalescence of numerous small veins from the vertebral venous plexus and from the musculature. The vein then courses inferiorly through the foramina transversaria, ending at the base of the neck in the brachiocephalic vein.

The Spinal Cord and Meninges. In the following dissection much of the intrinsic musculature of the

back will be reflected, and a laminectomy will be performed; that is, the vertebral laminae and spines will be excised, to expose the contents of the spinal canal. It may be desirable to retain one or more cadavers with the back musculature intact in the laboratory for later review of theses muscles.

Dissection. *As completely as possible, reflect or cut away the intrinsic back muscles from the spines and transverse processes of vertebrae T1 - L3. The ease with which subsequent procedures can be performed will be largely dependent upon the thoroughness with which you remove the intrinsic muscles from the vertebral column.*

Laminectomy. *With a saw, cut through the laminae longitudinally from T1 - L3. [A nearly total laminectomy is desirable, if time allows, for exposure of the spinal canal from C2 to the sacral hiatus; most of the spinal cord, spinal nerves and the subarachnoid space will be thereby revealed.]*

To facilitate the foregoing procedure the spines and laminae can be removed in segments of several successive vertebrae, after severing ligamentous attachments.

After excision of the vertebral laminae and spines, it may be that the vertebral canal is not exposed widely enough for clear visualization of its contents. If this is the case, remove additional bone as necessary with bone forceps or with mallet and chisel. Exercise particular care in the regions of the intervertebral foramina to avoid cutting or tearing away the spinal nerve rootlets.

*After the spinal canal has been opened, note the **extradural fat** and the **vertebral venous plexus** (Batson's veins). The fat within the **extradural space** may obscure the glistening surface of the spinal dura mater (from dura - tough, + mater - mother). The quantity of fat within the epidural space varies between individuals and it can also exist in varying degrees of liquefaction. The fat probably provides some measure of protection for the spinal cord.*

Remove the fat and the venous plexus from the epidural (or, extradural) space to clearly expose the dura mater.

The dura mater forms a tough, tubelike covering which is continuous cephalically with the inner layer of the dural covering of the brain. The dural sac ends caudally at about the level of the second sacral vertebra - on a plane which can be drawn between the posterior superior iliac spines. The dura mater continues from the end of the sac as a slender, tough connective tissue strand named the **filum of the dura mater**.

Incise the dura mater in the midline throughout its length with sharp scissors. Avoid incising the underlying arachnoid layer, if possible, by lifting and maintaining tension upon the dura mater. If the incision in the dura is made successfully, the arachnoid will appear as a thin, nearly transparent layer. If the arachnoid is accidentally cut, it can be peeled away from the internal surface of the dura with forceps.

*Identify the **subdural space**. Identify the **arachnoid meninx**. Incise the arachnoid membrane (Gk., arachne = spider) slightly to one side of the midline and identify the **subarachnoid space** and the **cerebrospinal fluid** - which pours out when the arachnoid is opened. Look for delicate, spiderweb-like strands which connect the inner surface of the arachnoid to the spinal cord. The subarachnoid space, like the subdural space, extends inferiorly to the level of the second sacral vertebra.*

*Identify the **spinal cord** and its covering of **pia mater** (Latin, pia - delicate + mater - mother). Look for the **denticulate ligament** on each side of the spinal cord. Lift it carefully with forceps for inspection, noting its toothlike serrations.*

Denticulations occur at the level of each vertebral pedicle, from the occipital bone - where the first denticulation is seen - to about the end of the spinal cord at the level of the body of L1. The attachment of the last denticulation to the dura is seen in the interval between the points of departure of the twelfth thoracic and first lumbar spinal nerves from the spinal canal - a useful clinical landmark. The denticulations pierce the arachnoid to attach to the dura. There are 21 pairs of denticulations.

At the caudal end of the spinal cord the pia mater continues as a strand of tissue, the **filum terminale** (specifically, the **filum terminale interna**). At the ending of the subarachnoid space caudally the filum terminale picks up coverings of arachnoid and dura; the filum then continues as the **filum terminale externa** to the dorsum of the coccyx.

*Observe the beginning of the filum terminale at its origin from the **conus medullaris**, the tapered end of the spinal cord. Note the cluster of large, nerve rootlets on either side of the conus medullaris which, because of their fancied resemblance to the tail of a horse, are referred to as the **cauda equina**. Observe the **lumbar enlargement** of the spinal cord.*

Confirm the following important facts: (1) The spinal cord terminates approximately at the level of the body of L1. (2) The subarachnoid and subdural spaces end at about the level of S2; that is, rather far inferior to the termination of the cord. (3) The level of S2 can be approximated by a line drawn through the posterior superior iliac spines. When one stands up, the posterior superior iliac spine is represented by a dimpling of the skin just above the buttock; when one bends forward at the waist, the bony prominence projects visible and is readily palpable.

There is also a cervical enlargement of the cord which extends from C4 to T1. These portions of the cord are visibly wider than other parts of the spinal cord because of the large numbers of neuronal cell bodies which they contain for the innervation of the upper and lower limbs, respectively.

*Again identify the **dorsal** and **ventral nerve rootlets**. In the cervical region the roots cross the subarachnoid space almost horizontally to their intervertebral foramina; but their passage becomes progressively more oblique through the thoracic and lumbar regions before the roots attain their respective foramina to exit the spine.* **Confirm that the denticulate ligaments lie between the dorsal and ventral rootlets of the spinal nerves.**

*With the bone pliers, break away enough bone of two adjacent vertebrae to observe the formation of a **spinal nerve** at an intervertebral foramen. Identify the **dorsal root ganglion** of the spinal nerve. At the level of the ganglion you will note that the dorsal and ventral roots are bound together tightly by their surrounding meningeal coverings. Secure and clean portions of the **dorsal primary ramus** and the **ventral primary ramus** of the spinal nerve.*

*By gently elevating the ventral primary ramus near its origin, attempt to identify one or two **communicating rami** leaving the deep (ventral) surface of the ramus. These communicating rami pass into the body cavity and connect to (or "communicate with") the sympathetic chains.*

*Inspect the surface of the spinal cord and attempt to identify the paired **dorsal spinal arteries**. Later, when a section of the spinal cord is removed, the **ventral spinal artery** will also be seen.*

*Upon an isolated segment of laminae and spines of several successive vertebrae, remove any obscuring tissues and identify the **supraspinous** and **interspinous** ligaments and the **ligamenta flava**. Note that the ligamentum flavum is present bilaterally, and connects the lamina of adjacent vertebrae.*

*Using a scalpel, expose and open the **fibrous capsule** of an **interarticular joint** (**zygapophyseal joint**). Note the smooth, **hyaline cartilage** covering of the articular facets. Move the **lumbar** and **sacral spinal nerve roots** aside in the upper lumbar portion of the vertebral canal, cut away any meninges which get in the way, and then identify the **posterior longitudinal ligament**, which passes along the dorsal aspects of the vertebral bodies and intervertebral disks, helping to bind them together. [The **anterior longitudinal ligament** lies upon the ventral aspects of the vertebral bodies and the disks.]*

The Spinal Cord and the Meninges. The central nervous system is covered by three membranous layers (Fig. 3:7), or meninges. The outermost

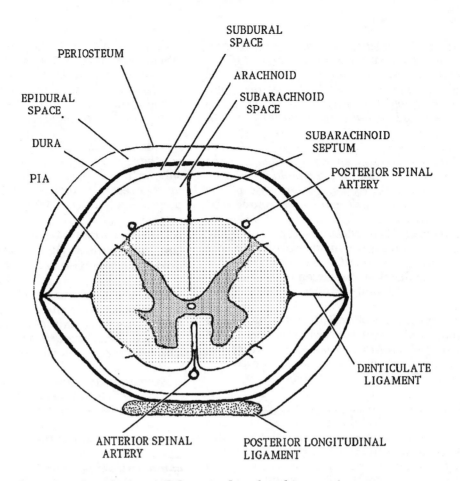

PERIOSTEUM

EPIDURAL SPACE

DURA

PIA

SUBDURAL SPACE

ARACHNOID

SUBARACHNOID SPACE

SUBARACHNOID SEPTUM

POSTERIOR SPINAL ARTERY

DENTICULATE LIGAMENT

ANTERIOR SPINAL ARTERY

POSTERIOR LONGITUDINAL LIGAMENT

Figure 3:7 Highly simplified schematic drawing of the spinal cord and its meninges.

covering is the dura mater, the middle layer is the arachnoid, and the third layer is the pia mater. The pia mater and arachnoid mater are referred to collectively as the **leptomeninges** *(lepto, Gk.= thin or weak)*. The dura mater is also called the **pachymeninx** *(pachys, Gk.= thick)*.

The space within the vertebral canal between the periosteum of the individual vertebrae and the dura mater is called the **epidural space** (or, **extradural** space). This space contains a variable quantity of fat and venous plexus, to which the eponym, "Batson's veins," has been applied. This venous plexus can be of clinical significance in the spread of disease processes. For instance,according to some authorities, prostatic or uterine cancer cells can invade pelvic veins and, by way of communicating vessels which pass through the ventral sacral foramina, enter the vertebral venous plexus. Subsequently the disease can spread to more superior parts of the body, including the brain.

The interval between the dura mater and the arachnoid is named the **subdural space**. The subdural space contains only a thin film of serous fluid. Normally, the dura mater and the arachnoid are in apposition with one another so that in reality no "space" intervenes between them.

The dura mater of the brain and spinal cord is supplied richly with sensory fibers by **meningeal branches** of cranial and spinal nerves. Excess pressure, tension, or inflammatory processes which affect the dura can cause intense pain.

Cerebrospinal Fluid. Internal to the thin, delicate arachnoid meningeal layer is the **subarachnoid space**, which contains the cerebrospinal fluid (CSF). The CSF is a clear, colorless fluid which provides protection for the brain and spinal cord, acting as a cushion between them and the bony skull and vertebral column. About 140 ml of CSF are present in the cranial and spinal subarachnoid spaces, although 500 ml are produced each 24 hr by special vessels (of the choroid plexus) in the ventricular system of the brain. Approximately 30 ml of fluid are present in the subarachnoid space of the vertebral canal, The CSF circulates slowly around the central nervous system and is reabsorbed back into the venous system of the head by way of specialized tufts of arachnoid which protrude into several of the dural venous sinuses which are present within the skull.

Development of Spinal Cord. Until the third month of intrauterine life, the spinal cord extends to the coccyx. At that stage, each spinal nerve can pass directly horizontally from its point of origin from the cord to its intervertebral foramen. Subsequently in development, however, the vertebral column grows at a rate which is much greater than that of the spinal cord. At the end of the fifth month the caudal end of the spinal cord is at the level of the superior end of the sacrum; by the time of birth, the termination of the spinal cord is at the level of the second lumbar vertebra or, variably, somewhat higher. In adults, the cord may extend to the disk between L1 and L2, although it can end somewhat higher, at the body of L1.

The spinal nerves below the cervical level must travel variably long courses within the vertebral canal to reach the foramina from which they exit. It is for this reason that below the level of the L1 vertebra the subarachnoid space is occupied by the cauda equina; it is composed of dorsal and ventral rootlets descending to their foramina. In effect, the specific spinal cord segment from which a pair of spinal nerves arises can be widely separated vertically from the intervertebral foramina through which those nerves leave the vertebral canal. Only the filum terminale and its coccygeal attachment remain to indicate the early relative length of the spinal cord and its attachment caudally.

Lumbar Puncture. The spinal fluid in the subarachnoid space can be sampled for study by insertion of a needle between vertebral laminae. Because the spinal cord ends near the lower aspect of the first lumbar vertebra, a needle can be introduced into the subarachnoid space with relative safety below the level of the second lumbar vertebra - preferably below the level of the third lumbar vertebra. This is most commonly done as a **lumbar puncture** between L3 and L4.

If a needle is inserted into the subarachnoid space below L3, cerebrospinal fluid can be safely withdrawn for study with relatively small likelihood of major injury to neural tissues. The needle enters the area of the cauda equina within the subarachnoid space, avoiding the spinal cord. Spinal anesthesia can be thus administered by injecting an appropriate agent into the subarachnoid space; similarly, radiopaque material can be injected for radiologic studies, as in myelograms of the spinal cord and spinal nerves.

The highest point reached by the iliac crests is at about the level of the fourth lumbar vertebra. Palpation of the crests bilaterally is useful in locating an appropriate and safe level for introduction of a needle into the subarachnoid space for anesthesia or myelography.

In contrast to spinal anesthesia, caudal anesthesia for more inferior nerve roots can be produced by placing the needle through the sacral hiatus into the epidural space. Such a procedure is not without risk, however; an improperly directed needle can pass through the sacrum by way of a ventral sacral foramen into pelvic organs. A baby **in utero** can be gravely injured in this way.

Blood Supply of the Spinal Cord. Two dorsal spinal arteries and one ventral spinal artery arise at

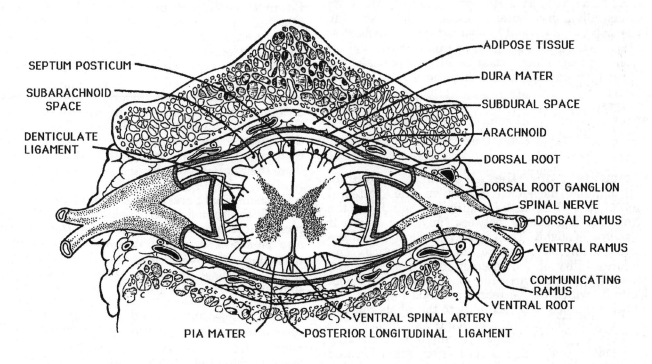

Figure 3:8 Semi-schematic drawing of a transverse section of the spinal cord and its coverings at the level of intervertebral foramina.

52

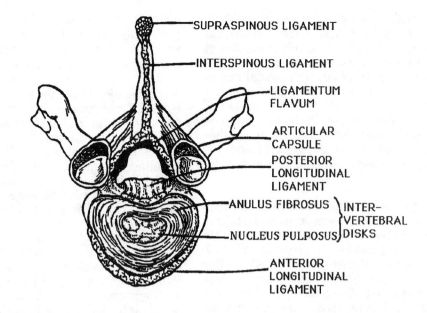

Figure 3:9 Intervertebral ligaments.

the level of the foramen magnum and pass to the spinal cord. Even casual inspection of these vessels reveals that they are of small caliber; in fact, these supply only the cervical extent of the cord. The arterial supply inferior to the cervical region is derived from reinforcing, **radicular arteries** which enter at each intervertebral foramen, passing inwards toward the spinal cord upon the spinal nerves and anastomosing longitudinally.

Radicular arteries arise, for the most part, from segmentally distributed vessels such as the intercostal arteries and lumbar arteries. The largest of these arteries is the "**great radicular artery**" (of Adamkiewicz), which arises usually on the left side between T6 and L3; it supplies the majority of the lumbosacral segments of the spinal cord. If the intercostal or lumbar artery from which this vessel arises is occluded, ischemia of a large segment of the spinal cord can occur.

Ligaments of the Vertebral Column. Considerable movement occurs in the vertebral column as a whole in the healthy individual; yet, the degree of movement between any two adjacent vertebrae is slight. The capacity for flexibility of the vertebral column is due to the slight elasticity and compressibility of the intervertebral disks and the innate laxity of the articular capsules of the synovial joints by which the vertebrae are held together. In addition to imparting flexibility to the whole column, the various ligaments and joints which join the vertebrae (Fig. 3:9) impart strength to resist the tremendous forces exerted in flexion, extension and rotation of the spine.

Ligamentous structures of the vertebral column include the following:

1. **supraspinous ligaments** - including the ligamentum nuchae
2. **interspinous ligaments**
3. **ligamenta flava**
4. **fibrous capsules of interarticular joints**
5. **anterior longitudinal ligament**
6. **posterior longitudinal ligament**
7. **intervertebral disks**

Communicating Rami. Every spinal nerve is attached to its ipsilateral (on the same side) sympathetic chain by a **gray communicating ramus**. This is a short, very slender nerve which carries postganglionic sympathetic fibers from a chain ganglion to the spinal nerve. The spinal nerve then distributes these sympathetic fibers by way of its ventral or dorsal primary ramus to blood vessels, sweat glands, pilomotor muscles of the body wall or the limbs. Gray communicating rami are nerves composed totally of **unmyelinated** axons, giving them their particular color.

Certain spinal nerves, specifically the first thoracic through the second lumbar spinal nerves, have gray communicating rami as described above, but each also possesses a **white communicating ramus**, consisting of **myelinated** axons. The myelin sheathes of these fiber, collectively, give the nerve a shiny, whitish appearance.

The spinal cord nucleus for preganglionic (primary) sympathetic neurons (the intermediolateral cell column - IML) is present at cord levels T1 to L2. The axons of these neurons leave the spinal cord by way of the ventral roots. They then pass through the spinal nerve trunk into the ventral primary ramus to reach the white communicating ramus. White

53

communicating rami carry the preganglionic sympathetic fibers from the spinal nerves T1 to L2 to the sympathetic chain. The preganglionic fibers synapse in the segmental ganglia, thus recruiting postganglionic fibers for sympathetic stimulation as noted above.

Note, then, that spinal nerves T1 to L2 have two communicating rami, one white and one gray, whereas each of the other spinal nerves has only a gray communicating ramus connecting it to the sympathetic chain.

The means by which sympathetic supply gets to the thoracic and upper lumbar spinal nerves is not difficult to perceive; but how is this achieved for cervical spinal nerves, lower lumbar, sacral and coccygeal nerves? In this way, simply: After reaching the sympathetic chains by white communicating rami, some preganglionic fibers ascend in the chain before synapsing; other such axons descend in the chain before synapsing with postganglionic neurons in ganglia at the levels of the other spinal nerves.

Questions for review and study

1. What is the innervation of the intrinsic muscles of the back?

Skeletal motor branches of dorsal primary rami

2. What is the vertebral canal?

The canal within the vertebral column formed by the vertebral foramina, within which the spinal cord lies

3. What passes through...
   a. vertebral foramina?
   b. intervertebral foramina?
   c. transverse foramina?

a. The spinal cord
b. The spinal nerves and small blood vessels which assist in supply of the spinal cord (radicular vessels)
c. The vertebral artery and the vertebral veins (through the transverse processes of C1 - C6)

4. Name the kinds of ligamentous structures which hold subjacent vertebrae together.

Supraspinous ligaments, ligamentum nuchae, interspinous ligaments, ligamenta flava, anterior longitudinal ligament, posterior longitudinal ligament, intervertebral disks, intertransverse ligaments, articular capsules of synovial joints between articular processes of the vertebrae.

5. What are the two portions of an intervertebral disk?

An outer, dense anulus fibrosus and an inner nucleus pulposus

6. What is the embryologic origin of the nucleus pulposus?

The embryologic origin is presumed to be the notochord.

7. What is the importance of the intervertebral disks? What type of joint does each form with the vertebrae which it joins together?

Their compressibility and elasticity allow the vertebral column to bend; they join the bodies of adjacent vertebrae; the inner portion of a disk can herniate and press upon the spinal cord or spinal nerves. The joint formed is called a symphysis and it is reinforced by the anterior and posterior longitudinal ligaments.

8. What is the ligamentum nuchae?

The supraspinous ligament in the cervical region, forming a thickened fibroelastic band connecting the base of the skull and the spines of the cervical vertebrae

9. What type of joint is formed between the superior articular processes of one vertebra with the inferior articular processes of an adjacent vertebra?

A synovial joint; that is, a rather freely moveable joint. Between vertebrae this movement is of a gliding nature.

10. What are the three major components of a synovial joint?

a. An outer fibrous articular capsule which holds the apposing bony surfaces together
b. An internally lining synovial membrane which secretes a slippery fluid into the joint cavity to facilitate movement
c. The opposing ends of the bones are covered with hyaline cartilage.

11. What are the primary curves of the vertebral column?

The thoracic and pelvic (sacrococcygeal) curves; "primary," because they are present in fetal life.

12. What are the secondary curves of the vertebral column?

The cervical and lumbar curves are often called compensatory curves; they are due, in part, to attaining upright posture and locomotion.

13. Name and define three abnormal curvatures of the vertebral column. ("Abnormal," when excessive)

Scoliosis = lateral curvature
Kyphosis = hunchback
Lordosis = swayback

14. What are the contents of the...
a. epidural space?
b. subdural space?
c. subarachnoid space?

a. Vertebral venous plexus and fat
b. A small amount of serous fluid
c. Cerebrospinal fluid (CSF)

15. At what vertebral level does the spinal cord terminate...
a. in the late embryonic period?
b. in the newborn?
c. in the adult?

a. At the end of the vertebral column
b. At, or about the level of the second lumbar vertebra (VL2). The vertebral column grows much faster and much longer than the spinal cord does.
c. At about the level of the disk between vertebra L1 and L2 or slightly higher (body of L1).

16. Where do the subdural and the subarachnoid spaces terminate inferiorly?

At the level of vertebral segment S2 of the sacrum, or the level of a line drawn between the two posterior superior iliac spines.

17. Where do the dura mater and the pia mater terminate inferiorly?

They terminate as the filum terminale externa at the coccyx.

18. What is the name of the fibrous bands that extend laterally from the pia mater to the dura between the dorsal and ventral nerve rootlets?

Denticulate ligaments

19. At what vertebral level does the last denticulation occur?

The L1 nerve roots lie upon the last process of the denticulate ligament at the level of vertebra L1.

20. Why is spinal anesthesia performed below vertebral level L3?

To avoid the spinal cord

21. Assuming a needle were placed directly in the midline, name in order the structures pierced before entering the subarachnoid space between VL3 and VL4.

Skin, fascia, supraspinous ligament, interspinous ligament, epidural tissues, dura, subdural space, arachnoid mater

22. Differentiate between the greater occipital nerve and the suboccipital nerve.

Greater occipital nerve = the medial branch of the dorsal primary ramus of C2. Suboccipital nerve = the dorsal primary ramus of C1.

23. Name the suboccipital muscles. Which of these help bound the suboccipital triangle? What is their innervation?

Suboccipital muscles: rectus capitis posterior major, obliquus capitis inferior, obliquus capitis superior, rectus capitis posterior minor. Only the first three of the four listed are considered to bound the triangle. Each is supplied by the suboccipital nerve.

24. What are the contents of the suboccipital triangle?

Contents: vertebral artery; dorsal primary ramus of C1 (suboccipital nerve); venous plexus; anastomosing small arteries

25. What is the most frequent defect in the development of the vertebral column?

Spina bifida - failure of the union between the two sides of a vertebral arch

26. What is the clinical significance of spina bifida?

The meninges can herniate from the vertebral canal = meningocele. The meninges and spinal cord can herniate together through the defect in the vertebral column = meningomyelocele

27. What is spondylolisthesis?

A slipping forward of a vertebral body; most commonly, a forward slipping of the body of VL5 over the sacrum, or of VL4 upon VL5.

28. What are the sources of arterial supply to the spinal cord?

a. Anterior spinal artery - two arise from the vertebral arteries and combine to form one median artery ventral to the cord.
b. Posterior spinal arteries - arise either from the vertebral arteries or from the posterior inferior cerebellar branches of the vertebral arteries. These two arteries pass longitudinally upon the posterolateral aspects of the spinal cord.
c. Radicular branches of the vertebral, ascending cervical, inferior thyroid, intercostal, lumbar, and lateral sacral arteries.

29. How long are the roots of spinal nerves?

The length of a nerve root depends upon the distance it must travel from the spinal cord to its exit from the vertebral canal. Cervical root C1 is several millimeters long; coccygeal roots can be more than 250 millimeters in length before they combine to form coccygeal spinal nerves.

30. Through what opening, and into what space does a needle pass for caudal anesthesia?

The needle passes through the sacral hiatus and into the epidural (extradural) space for anesthesia of the perineum and external genitalia

31. What vertebral level may be approximated by the highest (most superior) level reached by the iliac crests? In what way can this fact be applied clinically?

About L4, a relatively safe level for sampling CSF or performing spinal anesthesia.

32. What functional and structural features of spinal nerve C1 differentiate it from most other spinal nerves?

The first cervical spinal nerve has no cutaneous distribution. Both its dorsal and ventral primary rami carry mostly motor fibers to skeletal muscles; therefore, its dorsal root ganglia are typically very small, with sensory neuronal cell bodies only for specialized receptors associated with the muscles supplied.

LABORATORY IDENTIFICATION CHECK-LIST

The Spinal Cord and the Suboccipital Triangle

parts of typical vertebra
    vertebral body
    vertebral arch
    pedicles
    superior and inferior vertebral notches
    laminae
    spinous process
    transverse process
    superior and inferior articular processes
    zygopophyseal facets
    vertebral foramen

intervertebral foramen

thoracic vertebrae
    general vertebral characteristics
    costal facets, demi-facets

cervical vertebrae
    general vertebral characteristics
    foramen transversarium

atlas
    anterior arch
    posterior arch
    lateral masses
    sulcus for vertebral artery
    facet for articulation with dens
    facets for occipital condyles

axis
    spine
    odontoid process (dens)

lumbar vertebrae
    general vertebral characteristics

sacrum
    articular processes for VL5
    spinous processes
    sacral hiatus and cornua
    promontory
    ventral sacral foramina
    dorsal sacral foramina
    auricular surfaces
    alae of sacrum

greater occipital nerve
splenius muscle
semispinalis capitis muscle
obliquus capitis inferioris
obliquus capitis superioris
rectus capitis posterior major

rectus capitis posterior minor
suboccipital nerve
posterior atlanto-occipital membrane
vertebral artery

epidural fat
vertebral venous plexus
dura mater, subdural space
arachnoid mater, subarachnoid space
filum terminale interna
conus medullaris
cauda equina
lumbar enlargement of spinal cord

spinal nerve
dorsal root, dorsal root ganglion
ventral root
dorsal primary ramus, ventral primary ramus
communicating ramus

dorsal spinal arteries
ventral spinal artery

supraspinous ligament, ligamentum nuchae
interspinous ligament
ligamentum flavum
fibrous capsule of interarticular joint

posterior longitudinal ligament

DEFINITIONS

Ala (pl. alae) [L. "wing"]
A general term for a wing-like structure or process.

Arachnoid (pl. arachnoidea) [Gr. *arachnoeides* - like a cobweb]
Resembling a spider's web; a delicate membrane interposed between dura mater and the pia mater, being separated from the pia mater by the subarachnoid space.

Atlas [Gr. *Atlas,* the Greek god who bears up the pillars of heaven]
The first cervical vertebra, which articulates above with the occipital bone and below with the axis.

Axis (pl. axes) [Gr. *axon* axle]
A line about which a revolving body turns or about which a structure would turn if it did revolve; the second cervical vertebrae.

Cauda equina (pl. caudae) [L.*cauda,* a tail + *equus,* horse]
The collection of spinal roots that descend from the lower part of the spinal cord and occupy the vertebral canal below the cord; their appearance resembles the tail of a horse.

Dens (pl. dentes) [L. a tooth]
A tooth or toothlike structure.

Endosteum [Gr. *endo-* inside + *osteon* bone]
The tissue lining the medullary cavity of a bone or the cavities of the skull.

Facet [Fr. *facette,* little face]
A small plane surface on a hard body, as on a bone for articulation with other bones.

Foramen (pl. foramina) [L. an aperture or hole]
A natural opening or passage.

Hiatus [L. a gap or aperture]
A general term for a gap, cleft, or opening.

Kyphosis [Gr. *kyphosis* humpback]
Abnormally increased convexity in the curvature of the thoracic spine as viewed from the side; hunchback.

Lamina (pl. laminae) [L. a thin plate]
A thin flat plate or layer.

Laminectomy [L. *lamina* layer + Gr. *ektome* excision]
Excision of the posterior arch of a vertebra.

Leptomeninx (pl. leptomeninges) [Gr. *Leptos,* tender + *meninx,* membrane]
The pia mater and arachnoid considered together as one functional unit.

Ligamentum flavum (pl. ligamenta) [L. *flavus,* yellow]
Any of a series of bands of yellow elastic tissue attached to and extending between the ventral portions of the laminae of two adjacent vertebrae, from the junction of the axis and the third cervical vertebrae to the junction of the fifth lumbar vertebra and the sacrum.

Meningocele [Gr. *meningo,* membrane + *kele* hernia]
Hernial protrusion of the meninges through a defect in the skull or vertebral column.

Meningomyelocele [Gr. *meningo-* + *myelos,* marrow + *kele,* hernia]
Hernial protrusion of a part of the meninges and substance of the spinal cord through a defect in the vertebral column.

Meninx (pl. Meninges) [Gr. *meninx,* membrane]
A membrane; especially one of the three membranes enveloping the brain and spinal cord.

Pachymeninx (pl. pachymeninges) [Gr. *pachy,* thick, tough + *meninx,* membrane]
The dura mater, the outermost, tough covering of the spinal cord.

Pedicle [L. *pediculus,* a little foot]
A footlike, stemlike, or narrow basal part or structure.

Periosteum [Gr. *peri,* around + *osteon,* bone]
The membrane which intimately invests bone.

Rachischisis [Gr. *rach,* the spine + *schisis,* cleft]
Congenital fissure of the spinal column.

Scoliosis [Gr. *skoliosis,* twisted]
An appreciable lateral deviation in the normally straight vertical line of the spine.

Spina bifida - A developmental anomaly characterized by defective closure of the bony encasement of the spinal cord, through which the cord and meninges may or may not protrude.

Spondylolisthesis [Gr.*spondyl-* vertebra, + *olisthan-ein,* to slip]
> Forward displacement of one vertebra over another, usually of the fifth lumbar over the body of the sacrum, or the fourth lumbar over the fifth, usually due to a defect in the area of the lamina between the superior and inferior articular processes.

Spondylolysis [Gr. *spondylo-* vertebra, + *lysis,* dissolution]
> Separation of a vertebra.

Sulcus (pl. sulci) – A groove, trench, or furrow.

PART III

THE UPPER LIMB

CHAPTER 4: PECTORAL REGION AND BREAST

CHAPTER 5: THE DELTOID AND SCAPULAR REGIONS

CHAPTER 6: THE AXILLA AND BRACHIUM

CHAPTER 7: THE ANTEBRACHIUM

CHAPTER 8: THE HAND

CHAPTER 9: ARTICULATIONS OF THE UPPER LIMB

CHAPTER 4

PECTORAL REGION AND BREAST

The bony cage of the thorax is conical in shape, having its relatively narrow apex above (the superior thoracic aperture) and its base below (the inferior thoracic aperture). The superior aperture is packed rather tightly by structures passing between the thorax and neck including the trachea, esophagus, large blood vessels and nerves and the apical portions of the lungs. The inferior aperture of the thorax is closed by the muscular diaphragm.

Underlying the anterior aspect of the thoracic wall are several bony features which are helpful, palpable landmarks, particularly for localizing major features of the pectoral region. *Using Figure 4:1 as a guide, note the following landmarks with your fingertips upon yourself, classmates and the cadaver.*

1. The **suprasternal notch**.
2. The **sternal angle** (of Louis or Ludwig)
3. **Body** of the sternum

4. The *infrasternal notch*
5. *Xiphoid process of the sternum*

The **sternal angle** is formed by the junction of the manubrium and body of the sternum and marks the attachment of the **costal cartilages** of the second pair of ribs. As will be seen later, the sternal angle is an important topographical landmark, a palpable external point of reference to the location of numerous underlying visceral structures within the chest. Beginning at this point one may also count the ribs and the **intercostal spaces** between the ribs. In a small percentage of people, it is the third rib which articulates at the sternal angle.

Palpation. *Palpate the* **clavicle** *throughout its length, from the suprasternal notch to the tip of the shoulder. Identify the* **acromion process** *of the* **scapula**, *which forms the "tip" of the shoulder (akron-tip + omos-shoulder). Study all of the above features upon osteological material.*

A number of conventional reference lines can be drawn on the thoracic wall which are helpful in describing the topography of the chest and are used often in clinical practice. Among the more commonly used are the **midsternal, parasternal, mid-clavicular, anterior axillary, mid-axillary** and **posterior axillary** lines (Fig. 4:2).

The midsternal line connects the middle of the suprasternal notch with the **xiphisternal junction** or **infrasternal notch**. The parasternal line is usually thought of as a vertical line just lateral to the sternum. The midclavicular line in most people passes longitudinally just medial to the nipple.

The anterior axillary line is a vertical line which passes inferiorly from the **anterior axillary fold,** a prominent fold formed by skin and subcutaneous tissues over the underlying pectoral musculature. The posterior axillary line is associated in a similar way with the **posterior axillary fold** over the latissimus dorsi muscle. The midaxillary line is simply a longitudinal line equidistant between the anterior and posterior axillary lines on the side of the chest wall.

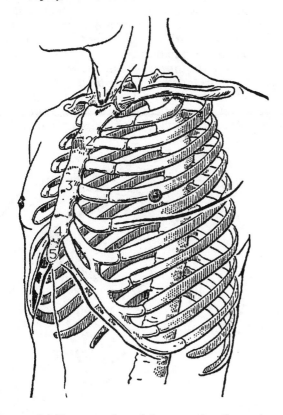

Figure 4:1 Topography of the anterior thoracic wall.

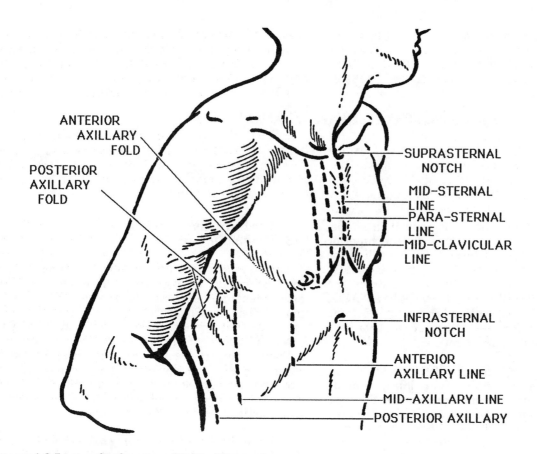

Figure 4:2 Lines of reference. Right oblique view.

ANTERIOR AXILLARY FOLD

POSTERIOR AXILLARY FOLD

SUPRASTERNAL NOTCH

MID-STERNAL LINE

PARA-STERNAL LINE

MID-CLAVICULAR LINE

INFRASTERNAL NOTCH

ANTERIOR AXILLARY LINE

MID-AXILLARY LINE

POSTERIOR AXILLARY

Dissection. *Reflection of Skin.* *Make a mid-sternal incision from the suprasternal notch to the infrasternal notch, and then make a horizontal incision which extends from the infrasternal notch to the mid-axillary line. Divide the skin over the clavicle to the tip of the shoulder (fig 4:3). This incision should then be extended distally upon the arm to a point approximately two inches above the elbow. An encircling incision about the arm will permit removal of the skin from the upper arm.*

Reflect and remove the skin from the thorax, shoulders, axillae and proximal portions of the arms.

*Subsequent to the removal of the skin, the superficial fascia can be readily reflected from the midsternal line to the midaxillary line by combined blunt and sharp dissection. As the superficial fascia is removed you may encounter **anterior cutaneous branches** of ventral primary rami and vessels emerging near the sternum. The vessels are the **perforating branches** of the internal thoracic artery and the **perforating tributaries** to the internal thoracic vein.*

During the reflection of fascia near the mid-axillary line, **lateral cutaneous branches of ventral primary rami** may be exposed where they enter the superficial fascia.

Dissection of the Mammary Gland. In the female cadaver the breast can be removed intact with the skin and superficial fascia of the pectoral region and then be examined further following the dissection of the underlying musculature. *Those who are dissecting male cadavers should take the time to observe the morphology of the breast of a female cadaver in the laboratory. Dissectors of the female are urged to assist their colleagues by pointing out salient features in the dissection of the mammary gland.*

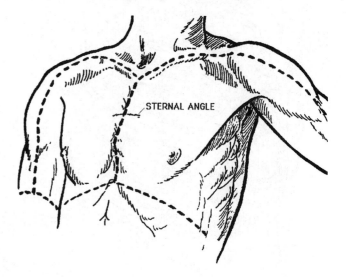

STERNAL ANGLE

Figure 4:3 Lines of incision.

This dissection will help you to understand the relationship of the breast to the pectoral region, as well as to better appreciate the clinical relationships of mastectomy (excision of breast tissues) to the anatomy of the region.

Topography. The **mammary gland** "normally" extends vertically from the second to the sixth rib and, laterally, from the side of the sternum to the mid-axillary line. The **areola** possesses numerous elevations, the **areolar glands** (of Montgomery), which aid in lubricating the nipple during lactation (def.: milk + to suckle.) During pregnancy the areola deepens in pigmentation.

The terms "mammary gland" and "breast" are not totally synonymous. The glandular elements are concealed for the most part by the contours of associated adipose and fibrous tissue and underlying musculature. In addition, the parenchymal tissues may extend to the midsternal line medially and deeply into the axilla laterally, hidden by the overlying anterior axillary fold. These parts of the gland can escape detection without very careful palpation and observation.

The **nipple** is situated typically at about the fourth intercostal space in both sexes. The topography of the breast is subject to variations due to the menstrual cycle, pregnancy, age and obesity.

Because of its location embryologically, the nipple receives its nerve supply from the fourth thoracic (or, intercostal) nerve. This fact is important surgically in breast reconstruction and other breast procedures.

Some fifteen to twenty lactiferous ducts pass radially from the nipple to a similar number of **lobes** of glandular tissue. The **lactiferous ducts** may possess an expanded part (the lactiferous sinus or ampulla) deep to the nipple. The ducts become very narrow as they pass through the tissue of the nipple, each terminating separately upon its surface. The secretory tissue is usually thickest in the areolar region.

*Palpate the **anterior axillary** fold and the **posterior axillary fold**. Observe by palpation whether there are extensions of the breast **parenchyma** (def.: distinguishing tissue of a gland or organ) into the axilla.*

Dissection. *In addition to the midsternal, clavicular and brachial (arm) incisions described in the removal of skin from the male, make an incision which encircles the areola. Lift the skin at the edge of the incision with your forceps. Separate some of the fatty tissue away from the skin with a probe while tensing the skin with the forceps. Note the **retinacula cutis**, which begin at the dermis and extend deeply into the breast, forming fibrous septae and irregular bands of dense connective tissue. Lift the skin of the areola and observe the retinacula cutis associated with it. In most aged cadavers, little will remain of the duct system or glandular tissue, being replaced simply by fibrous tissue infiltrated with fat.*

Posterior to the breast are the deep layer of the superficial fascia (membranous layer) and then the **retromammary space** (occupied by areolar tissue) and the deep fascia covering the pectoralis major and serratus anterior muscles. If cancer invades the retromammary space, its involvement of both the superficial fascia and the deep fascia covering the pectoralis major can result in fixation of the gland to the muscle, with consequent loss of the normal mobility of the breast.

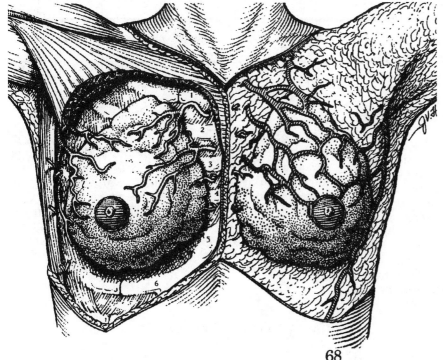

Figure 4:4 Blood supply of the breast. Veins shown on the left breast; arteries on the right breast.

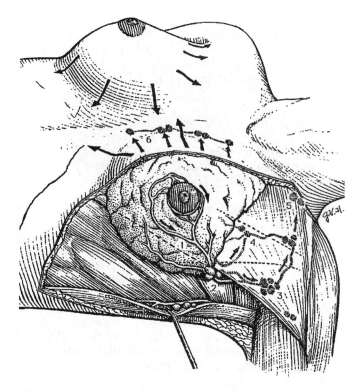

Figure 4:5 Lymph drainage of the breast. Directions of lymph flow from skin indicated by arrows on right breast and medial side of left breast. 1, Areolar plexus of vessels, draining areola, nipple and some parenchyma. 2, Pectoral nodes. 3, Central axillary nodes. 4, Interpectoral nodes (a path which can bypass central axillary nodes). 5, Apical, infraclavicular nodes. 6, Retrosternal nodes.

Blood Supply. The mammary gland is highly vascular, and is supplied by two or more **perforating branches** of the internal thoracic artery and by several branches of the axillary artery, especially the **lateral thoracic** and other, mammary branches. The venous drainage is provided by tributaries to the axillary, internal thoracic and intercostal veins. The intercostal veins provide direct communications with the vertebral plexus of veins. This is a route sometimes taken in the spread of a disease process such as cancer. It should be noted that the principal arteries supplying the breast are received above the level of the nipple (Fig. 4:4).

Nerve supply. The cutaneous areas of the breast just inferior to the clavicle receive their innervation by way of the supraclavicular nerves of the cervical plexus (C3, C4). Anterior and lateral cutaneous branches of ventral primary rami of spinal nerves T2-T6 supply most of the remainder of the breast region. The nipple is supplied by the fourth thoracic spinal nerve, especially by the lateral cutaneous branch of the ventral primary ramus. This branch leaves its intercostal space near the mid-axillary line and passes anteriorly to reach the areola and nipple.

Lymphatic Drainage. Lymphatic flow from most of the **glandular tissue** and from the **areola** and **nipple** passes first to the **anterior pectoral lymph nodes** beneath the lower border of the pectoralis major and along the lateral thoracic vein (Fig. 4:5). This lymph flows then to other axillary nodes and nodes located along the axillary vein. Lymph from these passes to the **infraclavicular** and **apical nodes** in the region of the infraclavicular fossa. See Figure 4:5 for the locations of principle node groups.

Lymph vessels from the medial aspect of the breast can carry lymph to retrosternal channels or communicate with lymph vessels of the opposite breast. Lymph from the medial side can course in an epigastric direction (below the infrasternal notch), spreading in some instances into lymphatics of the abdominal viscera.

The Pectoral Region

Dissection. *Identify the **pectoralis major muscle** (Fig. 4:6 - 8). The thin, tough fascia which invests this muscle is named the **pectoral fascia**. After cleaning the fascia from the pectoralis major, sever its costal, sternal and clavicular attachments and turn the muscle laterally to its insertion upon the humerus. **The clavicular portion of the pectoralis major must be transected with care to avoid cutting important vessels and nerves, including the lateral pectoral nerve.** [Note Figure 4:8.]*

Clean the pectoralis major thoroughly and note the manner in which its tendon twists upon itself as it passes to insertion. This is due to the fact that the inferior muscle fibers insert more proximally upon the humerus than do those which arise from the clavicle and manubrium (Fig. 4:6).

The pectoralis major arises from the sternum, the cartilages of the first seven ribs and from the medial half of the clavicle. The pectoralis major is separated from the deltoid muscle by the deltopectoral groove (Fig. 4:7). *Within the **deltopectoral groove**, covered by the pectoral fascia, lies the **cephalic vein**. This vein can be exposed by dividing the fascia which lies superficial to it.*

The **cephalic vein**, as will be seen later, begins upon the lateral side of the dorsum of the hand, and terminates by joining the axillary vein in the infraclavicular fossa (Fig. 4:8, 12), after piercing the infraclavicular fascia - the fascia which forms a floor for the infraclavicular fossa. The cephalic vein can serve as a collateral venous channel after occlusion of the axillary vein distally in the axilla. The cephalic vein is also a useful guide to the first part of the axillary artery.

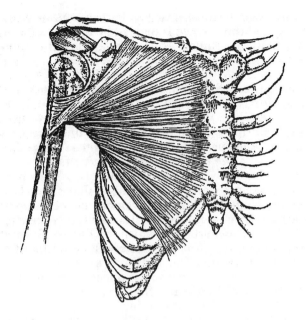

Figure 4:6 The pectoralis major and its attachments

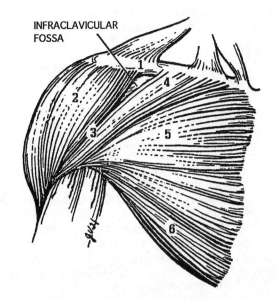

INFRACLAVICULAR FOSSA

Figure 4:7 Features of the pectoral region. 1, Clavicle. 2, Deltoid muscle. 3, Deltopectoral groove. 4, Pectoralis major - clavicular head. 5, Sternal head. 6, Costal head.

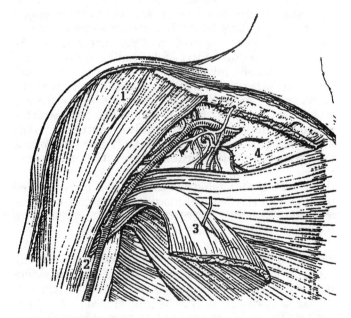

Figure 4:8 Exposure of the clavipectoral fascia. 1, Deltoid muscle. 2, Cephalic vein. 3, Clavicular head of pectoralis major with lateral pectoral nerve (cut). 4, Clavipectoral fascia.

*Turning aside the pectoralis major, observe the pectoralis minor, arising from the third, fourth and fifth ribs, passing to the coracoid process (def. coracoid: crow's beak) of the scapula, upon which it inserts (Fig. 4:9). Upon the deep surface of the pectoralis major identify the **lateral pectoral nerve** and **pectoral vessels**. Preserve these as the dissection proceeds. (Def. pectoral = pectus, breast bone)*

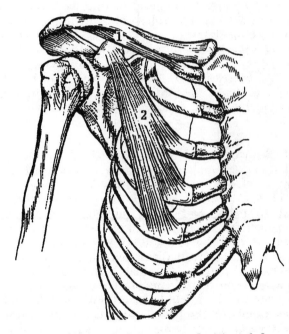

Figure 4:9 The subclavius muscle (1) and the pectoralis minor muscle (2) and their attachments.

*Between the clavicle and the upper border of the pectoralis minor identify the delicate **clavipectoral fascia** (Fig. 4:8). This fascia attaches proximally to the clavicle, beneath which it invests the small **subclavius muscle**. It then passes as a sheet toward the pectoralis minor, invests it, and then blends distally with the **axillary fascia**, there forming the so-called **suspensory ligament of the axilla** (Fig. 4:10). When the arm is abducted, the*

70

suspensory ligament produces the "hollow" in the axilla, because of the attachment of the fascia to the skin.

*Reflect the pectoralis minor from its origin. Observe the small branch or branches of the **medial pectoral nerve** which penetrate the pectoralis minor. A branch should be observed passing through the lateral, or inferior, border of this muscle to enter the pectoralis major.*

The **medial pectoral nerve** is so named because it arises from the **medial cord** of the **brachial plexus**, to be described later. The **lateral pectoral nerve** arises from the **lateral cord** of the **brachial plexus**. Because of a communication between the lateral and medial pectoral nerves after arising from the plexus, each nerve probably contributes to the innervation of both the pectoralis major and minor. Damage to the lateral pectoral nerve may selectively paralyze the clavicular part of the pectoralis major.

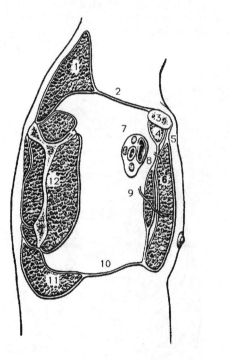

Figure 4:10 Parasagittal section through the pectoral region. 1, Trapezius muscle. 2, Cervical investing fascia. 3, Clavicle. 4, Subclavius muscle. 5, Pectoral fascia. 6, Pectoralis major. 7, Axillary sheath. 8, Lateral pectoral nerve, piercing clavipectoral fascia. 9, Medial pectoral nerve, entering pectoralis minor muscle. 10, Suspensory ligament of axilla. 11, Latissimus dorsi muscle. 12, Blade of scapula.

*Trace a **pectoral artery** to its origin from the **thoracoacromial artery** (Fig. 4:11), a branch of the axillary artery.* Branches of the thoracoacromial artery pass to the deltoid muscle, the acromion, the clavicle and to the pectoral muscles.

The clavipectoral fascia between the pectoralis minor and the clavicle is pierced by the cephalic vein, the thoracoacromial artery and vein, the lateral pectoral nerve and lymphatic vessels.

The Axillary Sheath. *Following the reflection of the pectoralis minor, the **axillary vein**, partially hidden by the axillary fascia, and the **axillary artery** can now be partially inspected. **Removal of the axillary fascia, however, should be deferred to a later time, when the axilla is completely dissected.***

The fascia observed about the axillary artery, the axillary vein and the large nerve elements of the brachial plexus is named the axillary sheath, a tube-like fascial tunnel which originates from the prevertebral fascia at the root of the neck. Injections can be made into the **axillary sheath** to induce anesthesia of the nerves to the upper limb (brachial plexus block), avoiding the problems which may accompany general anesthesia.

The Axillary Artery. The pectoralis minor muscle is an important "key" structure in the axillary region. The axillary artery is topographically divided into three parts by it (Fig. 4:11, 12). From the **first part**, proximal to the pectoralis minor, arises one vessel: the **supreme thoracic artery**, which supplies muscles of the first one or two **intercostal spaces**.

From the **second part** of the axillary artery, deep to the pectoralis minor, arise the **thoracoacromial** and the **lateral thoracic arteries**. The **third portion** of the axillary artery gives origin to the **anterior** and **posterior humeral circumflex arteries** and the **subscapular artery**. The subscapular artery divides almost immediately into the **scapular circumflex** and **thoracodorsal** arteries. The identification of the branches of the third part of the axillary artery should be deferred until the dissection of the axilla. *Identify and trace out the supreme thoracic, lateral thoracic and thoracoacromial arteries, if they are not yet exposed.*

Serratus Anterior. *Identify the **serratus anterior muscle** and its motor nerve, the **long thoracic nerve** (C5, 6, 7), which travels in the midaxillary line on the superficial surface of the muscle. Note the digitations of the serratus anterior and the emergence of the **lateral cutaneous nerves** between these digitations and those of the external oblique muscle of the abdomen. The serratus anterior arises from the upper eight ribs and inserts upon the vertebral border of the scapula.*

Intercostobrachial Nerve. *With the pectoralis minor reflected identify the **intercostobrachial nerve** (T2) emerging from the second intercostal space.* This nerve is sensory to the axilla and the upper medial aspect of the arm. In some specimens the third intercostal nerve may communicate with it.

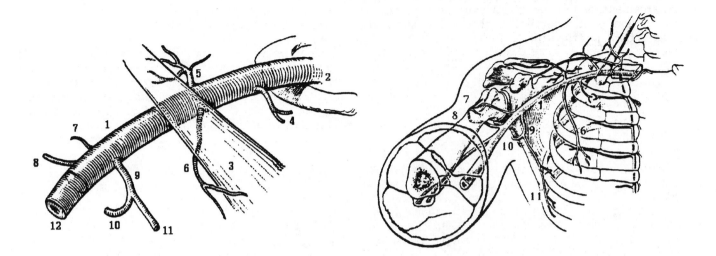

Figure 4:11 The axillary artery and its relations. 1, Axillary artery. 2, Subclavian artery. 3, Pectoralis minor. 4, Supreme thoracic artery. 5, Thoracoacromial artery. 6, Lateral thoracic artery. 7, Anterior humeral circumflex artery. 8, Posterior humeral circumflex artery. 9, Subscapular artery. 10, Circumflex scapular artery. 11, Thoracodorsal artery. 12, Brachial artery.

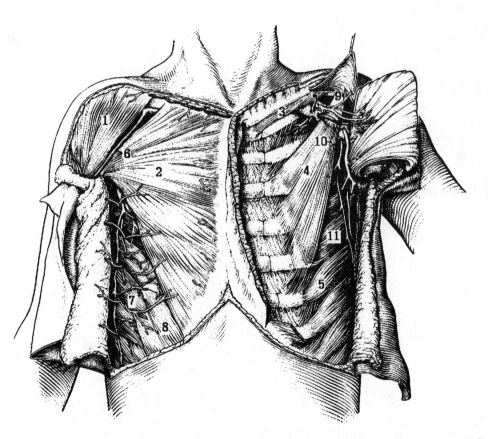

Figure 4:12 Muscles, nerves and vessels of the pectoral region. 1, Deltoid. 2, Pectoralis major. 3, Subclavius. 4, Pectoralis minor. 5, Serratus anterior. 6, Cephalic vein. 7, Lateral cutaneous nerves. 8, External oblique. 9, Lateral pectoral nerve and thoracoacromial vessels. 10, Medial pectoral nerve. 11, Long thoracic nerve.

72

The intercostobrachial nerve passes close enough to some of the axillary lymph nodes that their enlargement, as in cancer, may cause intense pain in the region of distribution of this nerve along the medial border of the arm.

TABLE 4:1 The Muscles of the Pectoral Region.

MUSCLES	ATTACHMENTS	FUNCTIONS	INNERVATION
Pectoralis Major	Origin: The sternum, the cartilages of the first seven ribs and the medial half of the clavicle. Insertion: Crest of the greater tubercle of the humerus (lateral lip of bicipital groove).	Flexes, adducts and rotates the arm medially. The clavicular part draws the arm or shoulder upward, forward or medialward. The sternocostal part draws the arm or shoulder forward, medialward and downward.	Medial and lateral pectoral nerves — fibers from the fifth, sixth, seventh, eighth cervical and the first thoracic nerves. **Clavicular head** by lateral pectoral only: fifth and sixth cervical nerves.
Pectoralis Minor	Origin: ribs 3-5. Insertion: Coracoid process of the scapula.	Protracts and depresses the scapula (draws it forward and downward); rotates it laterally. Raises the third, fourth and fifth ribs in forced inspiration.	Medial and lateral pectoral nerves; fibers from the fifth cervical to first thoracic nerves.
Subclavius	Origin: Cartilage of first rib. Insertion: Underside of the clavicle.	Depresses the clavicle slightly. [Protects the axillary artery in event of clavicular fracture.]	Nerve from the upper trunk of the brachial plexus—fibers from the fifth and sixth cervical nerves.
Serratus Anterior	Origin: Fleshy digitations of the upper eight ribs. Insertion:Vertebral border of scapula.	Protracts the scapula (draws it forward); the upper part of the muscle rotates the glenoid cavity of the scapula downward; the lower part of the muscle rotates the scapula upward, as when the arm is abducted above the level of the shoulder.	Long thoracic nerve — fibers from the fifth,sixth and seventh cervical nerves.

QUESTIONS FOR REVIEW AND STUDY

1. What is the sternal angle of Lewis?

The angle formed by the junction of the manubrium (def.: handle) and body of the sternum

2. What ribs articulate at the sternal angle?

Most commonly, the second pair of ribs, by their costal cartilages

3. What portion of the sternum lies just proximal to the epigastric fossa of the anterior abdominal wall?

The xiphoid (def.: swordshaped) process

4. What vertical reference line lies mid-way between the anterior and posterior axillary folds?

The mid-axillary line

5. What nerves enter the superficial fascia at the mid-axillary line?

The lateral cutaneous branches of the ventral primary rami

6. What nerves enter the superficial fascia at the lateral borders of the sternum?

The anterior cutaneous branches of the ventral primary rami

7. What name is given to ventral primary rami which pursue a course between the ribs from the intervertebral foramina to the sternum?

Intercostal nerves

8. What function is performed by intercostal nerves in addition to giving origin to lateral and anterior cutaneous nerves?

They innervate the intercostal muscles.

9. What vessels accompany the intercostal nerves? What is the origin of these arteries?

The intercostal arteries and veins. Most intercostal arteries arise from the aorta. Other sources include the costocervical trunks and the internal thoracic arteries.

10. What muscles form the anterior axillary fold?

The pectoral muscles

11. What muscle forms the posterior axillary fold?

The latissimus dorsi

12. What is the usual position of the nipple with respect to the thoracic wall?

In the fourth intercostal space

13. What is the normal extent of the breast?

From second to sixth ribs, vertically, and from the sternum to the mid-axillary line, with a prolongation upward into the axilla - the axillary tail.

14. What is the "milk line"?

A topographic line from the axilla to the groin along which supernumerary breasts may develop in male or female, usually manifested only as an extra nipple. Such "extra" breasts may be functional.

15. To what structures do the suspensory ligaments (of Cooper) attach?

The suspensory ligaments of the breast extend from the dermis to the deep membranous layer of the superficial fascia. They also attach to glandular elements.

16. How does peau d'orange (orange peel appearance) occur, with respect to the skin covering the breast?

Blockage of lymphatics which drain the skin results in subcutaneous edema. There appears to be "pitting" of the skin around each hair follicle, because the hair follicles attach to the subcutaneous tissue and the surrounding skin is edematous.

17. What is the cause of "dimpling", often seen in cancer of the breasts?

Contraction of the retinaculae of the breast (Cooper's ligaments), which attach to the dermis of the skin and to the parenchyma and milk ducts.

18. What is the cause of the lack of mobility of some cancerous breasts?

Fixation of the breast to underlying deep fascia and/or muscle by invasive disease.

19. What is the name of the potential space deep to the breast?

The retromammary space

20. How many openings are there in the nipple?

As many openings as lactiferous ducts; there are as many ducts as there are lobes (15-20).

21. What are the sources of blood supply to the breast?

Internal thoracic arteries, lateral thoracic artery, mammary branches of axillary, intercostal arteries

22. What are the first principal nodes encountered by lymph from the areola and nipple?

Anterior pectoral nodes beside the lateral thoracic vessels beneath the pectoralis minor.

23. Name five sites to which lymph from the breast may flow.

Axillary nodes, retrosternal nodes, lymphatics of opposite breast, directly to apical nodes, lymphatics of abdomen.

24. Give the boundaries of the deltopectoral triangle.

Deltoid, pectoralis major, clavicle

25. What structures lie within the deltopectoral groove?

Cephalic vein, deltoid branch of thoracoacromial artery.

26. To what bones do the pectoralis major and minor, respectively, pass to insertion?

Pectoralis major, humerus; pectoralis minor, coracoid process of scapula

27. What is the innervation of the pectoral muscles?

Medial and lateral pectoral nerves

28. What fascia covers the pectoralis major?

Pectoral fascia

29. What fascia passes from the clavicle to ensheath the pectoralis minor?

Clavipectoral fascia

30. Why is the lateral pectoral nerve so named, when it appears to lie medial to the medial pectoral nerve?

Because it is not named according to its position, but by its origin from the lateral cord of the brachial plexus; the medial pectoral nerve arises from the medial cord of plexus.

31. What is the source of blood supply to the pectoral muscles?

Pectoral branches of the thoracoacromial, lateral thoracic, intercostal arteries

32. What structures pierce the clavipectoral fascia superior to the upper border of the pectoralis minor muscle?

Cephalic vein, thoracoacromial artery and vein, lateral pectoral nerve, lymphatics

33. What is the one branch of the first part of the axillary artery?

The supreme (highest) thoracic artery

34. What are the two branches of the second part of the axillary artery?

The thoracoacromial and lateral thoracic

35. What are the three branches of the third part of the axillary artery?

The anterior and posterior humeral circumflex arteries and the subscapular artery

36. Matching. To the left of each muscle, place the letter which most correctly indicates its source of motor innervation.

1) _____Trapezius
2) _____Latissimus dorsi
3) _____Erector spinae
4) _____Transversospinalis
5) _____Posterior superior and inferior serrati
6) _____Serratus anterior
7) _____Intercostal muscles
8) _____Suboccipital muscles
9) _____Pectoralis major
10) _____Pectoralis minor

a. Greater occipital nerve (C2)
b. Suboccipital nerve (C1)
c. Medial and lateral pectoral nerves
d. Dorsal primary rami
e. Thoracodorsal nerve
f. Ventral primary rami
g. Cranial nerve XI, spinal accessory
h. Long thoracic nerve
i. Intercostal nerves

1) g
2) e
3) d
4) d
5) f
6) h
7) i
8) b
9) c
10) c

37. Which of the nerves listed above....

1.) Has no cutaneous distribution, although other such nerves do?

1) b

2.) Provides sensory branches to the skin of the scalp?

2) a

3.) Provides sensory branches to the skin by the sternum.?

3) i

4.) Provides sensory branches to the skin in the midaxillary line?

4) i

5.) Arise from the brachial plexus?

5) c,e,h

6.) Exits a foramen of the skull, rather than an intervertebral foramen?

6) g

7.) Are really ventral primary rami, but are not associated with the brachial plexus?

7) i

LABORATORY IDENTIFICATION CHECK-LIST

Breast and Anterior Thoracic Wall

To be palpated:

suprasternal notch
infrasternal notch
xiphoid process
body of sternum
sternal angle
clavicle
acromion process

On Skeleton: all of above, plus: manubrium, costal cartilages and coracoid process

On cadaver:

anterior axillary fold
posterior axillary fold
anterior cutaneous branches of intercostal nerves

lateral cutaneous branches of intercostal nerves
areola and areolar glands
nipple

suspensory ligaments of the breast

retromammary space

pectoralis major

pectoral fascia (muscular fascia of pectoralis major)
deltoid muscle
deltopectoral groove
cephalic vein

lateral pectoral nerve
pectoral artery and vein
clavipectoral fascia
subclavius muscle
axillary fascia (deep fascia)
suspensory ligament of axilla
pectoralis minor
medial pectoral nerve
lateral thoracic artery
thoracoacromial artery

axillary artery
axillary vein
axillary sheath
supreme thoracic artery
serratus anterior muscle
long thoracic nerve
intercostobrachial nerve

DEFINITIONS

Ampulla (pl. ampullae) [L. "a jug"]
A general term used to designate a flasklike dilation of a tubular structure.

Circumflex [L. *circumflexa,* bent about]
Curved like a bow.

Lactiferous [L. *lac ,* milk + *ferre,* to bear]
Producing or conveying milk.

Nipple - The pigmented projection on the anterior surface of the mammary gland, surrounded by the areola.

Parenchyma [Gr. "anything poured in beside"]
The essential elements of an organ.

Polymastia [Gr. *poly-* many + *mastos,* breast]
The presence of more than one pair of mammae, or breasts.

Polythelia [Gr. *poly-* many + *thele,* nipple + *-ia*]
The condition of having more than one pair of nipples.

Retinacula cutis (pl. retinaculum) [L. "a rope, cable"]
Bands of connective tissue attaching the corium to the subcutaneous tissue.

Retromammary - behind the mammary gland.

CHAPTER 5

DELTOID AND SCAPULAR REGIONS

Introduction. Some of the features of the deltoid and scapular regions may have been exposed previously, in the dissections of the back and pectoral regions. These structures should be reviewed and studied with care in this dissection.

Osteology and Superficial Anatomy

The dissection of the upper limb should be accompanied by frequent reference to the bony skeleton and illustrations in atlases. It should be performed bilaterally, so that one side of the specimen can later be used for study of the joints.

Palpate the **sternoclavicular joints** *upon yourself - at rest and in movement of the joints - and the* **acromion process, clavicle, spine of the scapula, medial** *and* **lateral humeral epicondyles** *and the* **olecranon** *(Fig. 5:1, 2). Can you palpate the coracoid process in the infraclavicular fossa? Try elevating one arm and hand above your head and deeply palpating in the infraclavicular fossa of that limb while elevating it, circumducting it and bringing it back to the anatomic position.*

Dissection. *Divide the skin over the* **cephalic vein** *from the deltopectoral groove to the wrist.* In some individuals the cephalic vein terminates by entering the vascular bed of the deltoid muscle, so that little can be seen of the cephalic vein in the deltopectoral groove. This vein is comparable in position and development to the great saphenous vein of the lower member. The great saphenous vein begins at the medial aspect of the foot and passes up the medial side of the lower limb and terminates superiorly at the femoral vein.

Make circumferential skin incisions at the wrist and proximal to the elbow and reflect the skin from the brachium and antebrachium, leaving the superficial fascia intact, for the time being.

Identify the **cephalic, basilic** *and* **median cubital veins** *and observe their* **superficial** *and* **deep perforating tributaries** *(Fig. 5:3, 4).* The basilic vein is comparable to the small (lesser) saphenous vein of the lower limb. That vein begins on the lateral aspect of the foot and ankle and passes upward to the soft hollow behind the knee, where the short saphenous vein drains into the popliteal vein.

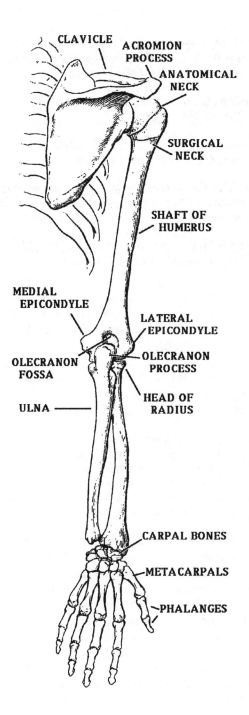

Figure 5:1 Posterior view of the bones of the upper limb

82

It can be noted in this context that in late fetal development the upper and lower limbs undergo gradual rotation in opposite directions.

The elbow and the knee point in the same direction early on in development. What is the "front" of the thigh in the anatomic position is developmentally the posterior aspect of the lower limb - the muscles there (for example, the quadriceps femoris) are supplied by posterior divisions of spinal nerves. When a child first begins to attempt to walk, the knees still point somewhat laterally, making the child appear bow-legged. Only later do the lower limbs complete their medial rotation so that the knees point forward.

The cephalic and basilic veins arise from the lateral and medial aspects, respectively, of the dorsal venous arch of the hand. The cephalic vein terminates, after traversing the deltopectoral groove, by piercing the pectoral and clavipectoral fascia and joining the axillary vein. The basilic vein ascends the medial aspect of the extremity, penetrating the deep fascia about half-way up the brachium. Thereafter the basilic vein joins the venae comitantes of the brachial artery, thereby forming the axillary vein. The cephalic and basilic veins are usually connected anterior to the elbow by the median cubital vein. The median cubital vein also receives deep communicating tributaries from deep veins of the antebrachium (forearm).

*Study Figures 5:3 and 4 to assist you in identifying the **posterior antebrachial cutaneous, medial antebrachial cutaneous** and the **lateral antebrachial cutaneous nerves** as they emerge from the deep fascia. The sources of these three nerves will be found in a later dissection.*

The posterior antebrachial cutaneous nerve arises from the radial nerve, the nerve which supplies the extensor compartments of the arm and forearm. The medial antebrachial cutaneous nerve arises from the medial cord of the brachial plexus, often in common with the medial brachial cutaneous nerve. The lateral antebrachial cutaneous nerve is the terminal branch of the musculocutaneous nerve, the nerve which supplies the muscles of the flexor compartment of the arm (the biceps brachii, for example).

Observe the proximity of the three cutaneous nerves relative to frequently utilized injection sites. Then, carefully, remove all superficial fascia from the upper limb from the shoulder to wrist, preserving the larger veins and cutaneous nerves. Observe that the medial antebrachial cutaneous nerve pierces the deep fascia of the arm together with the basilic vein. This fact is

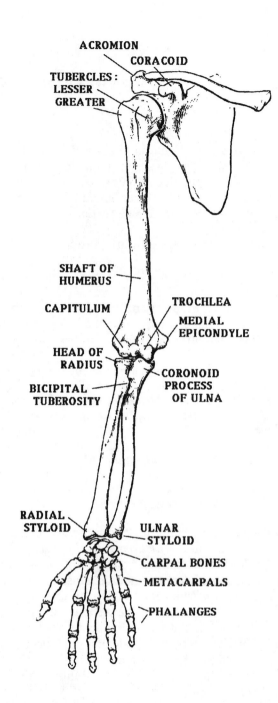

Figure 5:2 Anterior view of the bones of the upper limb.

important in clinical procedures such as elevating the basilic vein to a position just deep to the skin for use in dialysis. Cutting the medial antebrachial cutaneous nerve in the process, or entrapping it in sutures or scar, needs to be avoided.

Deltoid Region

Deltoid Muscle. *Identify the deltoid muscle. Define its borders and the orientation of its fibers by freeing the muscle of its fascial investment. The deltoid arises from the lateral third of the clavicle and the*

83

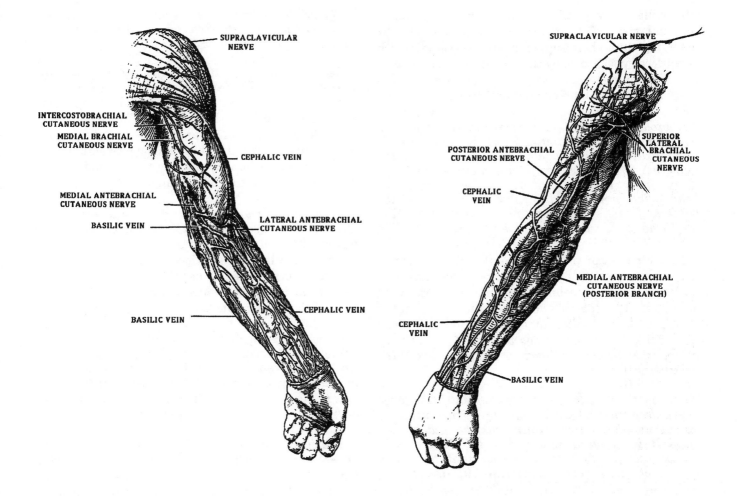

Figure 5:3 Superficial features of the flexor surface of the upper limb.

Figure 5:4 Superficial features of the extensor surface of the upper limb.

acromion process and spine of the scapula. Note the convergence of its fibers toward the deltoid tuberosity of the humerus. The deltoid is the principal abductor of the arm. Its anterior and posterior fibers, respectively, assist in flexion and extension of the arm. The deltoid is innervated by the axillary nerve from C5 and C6 (primarily C5).

Using a scalpel and scissors, reflect the anterior border of the deltoid laterally, dividing its attachment to the clavicle and acromion process. Continue reflecting the muscle laterally and posteriorly until the surgical neck of the humerus is visible, but leaving the deltoid muscle attached to the deltoid tuberosity.

As the deltoid muscle is turned aside, note its proximity to the underlying tendon of insertion of the pectoralis major and the position of the biceps brachii. Identify the long head and short head of the biceps.

Axillary Nerve. The axillary nerve supplies the teres minor and deltoid muscles and distributes sensory fibers to the skin overlying the deltoid muscle. The axillary nerve consists primarily of fibers from the C5 spinal nerve, as do several other nerves which supply muscles in the shoulder region. The cutaneous supply of the skin over the deltoid and the lateral aspect of the arm is derived from spinal nerve C5. In a lesion of the fifth cervical nerve (as from a herniated cervical disk or cervical spondylitis), there may be anesthesia of this area, in addition to associated muscular problems. See Figures 6:7-10 for illustrations of the dermatomes of the upper limb.

Identify the axillary nerve as it appears posterior to the surgical neck of the humerus (Fig. 5:5). The nerve is accompanied by the **posterior humeral circumflex artery**, *a branch of the third portion of* the axillary artery. The axillary nerve and posterior humeral circumflex artery appear in the field by emerging through the **quadrangular space**, which is bordered posteriorly by the long head of the triceps, the teres minor and teres major muscles and the surgical neck of the humerus (Fig. 5:8).

Thoroughly clean the axillary nerve and the posterior humeral circumflex vessels at their entrance into the deltoid muscle behind the surgical neck of the humerus. Protect them as you clean connective tissue away from the muscles which help form the boundaries for the quadrangular space. Review the borders of this space: teres major, teres minor, the long head of the triceps brachii, humerus.

How far inferior (in centimeters) to the tip of the acromion process does the axillary nerve make its appearance from behind the humerus in your specimen? It is easy to understand the importance of this fact as it applies to intramuscular injections here. *Look for the cutaneous branch of the axillary nerve, the* **upper (superior) lateral brachial cutaneous nerve.**

Bursae. *As the deltoid is reflected, identify the large bursa deep to it which, because of its two principal extensions, is called rather interchangeably the* **subdeltoid** *or* **subacromial bursa.** *Dissect away the connective tissue of the bursa until the heavy fibers of the* **coracoacromial ligament** *are well-delineated. Note the sharp lateral border of the coracoacromial ligament.* The tendon of the supraspinatus muscle is subject to inflammation or erosion where it passes beneath this edge of the ligament - sometimes necessitating surgical excision of the ligament to ensure long term relief from the problem.

Clean the insertion of the **pectoralis minor muscle** *and the origins of the* **coracobrachialis muscle** *and the* **short head of the biceps brachii** *at the coracoid process.*

The Scapular Region

Review. *Place the cadaver in the prone position. Review the attachments of the* **trapezius muscle.** It arises from the base of the skull, the ligamentum nuchae in the cervical region and from the spines of the thoracic vertebrae. From this broad origin the fibers of the trapezius pass to the lateral third of the clavicle and to the acromion and spine of the scapula. What is the innervation of the trapezius? You should remember that the trapezius and the sternocleido-mastoid muscles are both supplied by the spinal accessory nerve.

The origin of the trapezius should now be divided, if this has not already been done, and its neural and vascular supply should be cleaned.

Deep to the trapezius re-identify the **levator scapulae, rhomboideus minor** *and* **rhomboideus major muscles.** The levator scapulae inserts upon the superior angle of the scapula. The rhomboideus minor inserts superior to, and at the root of the spine of the scapula. The rhomboideus major inserts on the medial scapular border, inferior to the spine of the scapula, and upon the inferior angle of the scapula.

Transect the rhomboids at their vertebral origin. Upon their deep surface identify the **dorsal scapular nerve.** This nerve innervates the rhomboids and the levator scapulae (in addition to rami from C3 and C4). The dorsal scapular nerve arises from C5, one of the two motor nerves which arise directly from the roots of the brachial plexus.

Remove any obscuring fascia, areolar and adipose tissue and demonstrate the **omohyoid, supraspinatus, infraspinatus, teres minor** *and* **teres major muscles** *(Fig. 5:6). Cut the attachments of the trapezius to the spine and acromion process of the scapula, as necessary, to expose the deeper muscles.*

The omohyoid originates from the superior border of the scapula, medial to the scapular notch. This notch is bridged by the transverse scapular ligament. The omohyoid inserts upon the hyoid bone.

Suprascapular Artery and Nerve. *Trace the suprascapular artery from its origin to its crossing of the* **transverse scapular ligament** *to enter the supraspinous fossa, deep to the supraspinatus muscle (Fig. 5:6). Identify and clean the* **supraspinatus muscle** *and then, beginning medially, reflect the muscle laterally from the supraspinous fossa far enough to expose the* **suprascapular nerve and artery.** *Identify the* **infraspinatus muscle** *and reflect it laterally from the infraspinous fossa toward its humeral insertion.*

Note the passage of the suprascapular nerve and vessels around the **great scapular notch** *(Fig. 5:6, 7), where they enter the infraspinatus muscle. Trace the* **suprascapular nerve** *from its origin from the upper trunk of the brachial plexus (C5 and C6) to its passage deep to the transverse scapular ligament to enter the supraspinatus.* The suprascapular nerve innervates both the supraspinatus and infraspinatus muscles, primarily with fibers from the C5 spinal nerve level.

After its origin from the supraspinous fossa, the supraspinatus muscle passes beneath the coracoacromial ligament to reach the greater tubercle of the humerus, where it inserts. As noted before, the supraspinatus tendon can be irritated, worn away or torn where it contacts the sharp lateral edge of the ligament in   abduction of the limb.   This can obviously be a serious problem, especially in serious (or professional) athletes who must throw or swing powerfully in various sports.

It is said commonly that the supraspinatus is required for the first 15 degrees of abduction of the arm from the anatomic position.   It functions little, or not at all as a lateral rotator of the arm.   The deltoid assumes the role of principal abductor from 15 to 90 degrees. After the limb has been elevated to the level of the shoulder, other shoulder muscles (the trapezius and serratus anterior, in particular) rotate the scapula upward so that the limb can be elevated above the horizontal.   The tendon of the supraspinatus is probably even more important in that, because of its course over the head of the humerus, it assists in preventing upward dislocation of the head of the humerus from the shoulder joint.

If the innervation of the supraspinatus is interrupted, abduction of the extremity can be awkward. Following paralysis of the deltoid, upward rotation of the scapula together with the humerus can be effected by using the trapezius, serratus anterior and smaller muscles such as the levator scapulae and rhomboids in such a way that a patient can learn to compensate for deltoid loss, being able to abduct the limb to an overhead position, although with less strength.

The Rotator Cuff. The tendons of insertion of the supraspinatus, infraspinatus and teres minor muscles form the external, or lateral portion of the muscular "rotator cuff" of the shoulder in their collective passage about the capsule of the shoulder joint and insertion upon the greater tubercle of the humerus. This tendinous portion of the rotator cuff is subject to damage in common, often highly debilitating tears (which can quickly end a professional career in sports). With aging, there is in many individuals a gradual reduction in vascular supply to these tissues - increasing the likelihood of injuries which heal only slowly and often poorly.

The infraspinatus and teres minor are very important, along with the deltoid, in acting to

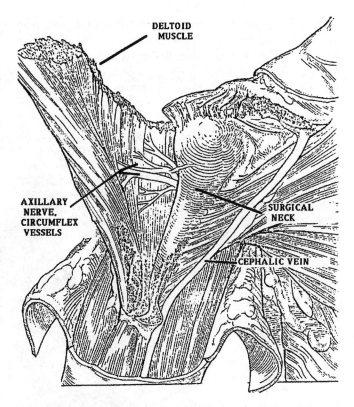

Figure 5:5 Axillary nerve and posterior humeral circumflex vessels - relation to surgical neck of humerus.

laterally rotate the arm at the shoulder joint. The subscapularis, the medial component of the rotator cuff, is the principal medial rotator of the shoulder. The significance of the cuff will be referred to again in a subsequent dissection.

The teres major is innervated by the lower subscapular nerve, a nerve which arises from the posterior cord of the brachial plexus (to be seen in the next dissection). The deltoid and teres minor muscles are supplied by the axillary nerve, which also arises from the posterior cord.

The **latissimus dorsi** muscle arises primarily from the spines of the vertebrae from T6 to the upper sacral region and the iliac crest. The tendon of the latissimus passes to the medial side of the humerus to insert into the floor of the bicipital groove, adjacent to the tendon of the teres major. The latissimus dorsi receives its nerve supply from the thoracodorsal nerve (or, middle subscapular nerve) from the posterior cord of the brachial plexus. This muscle extends, adducts and medially rotates the humerus.

Reflect the latissimus laterally from its origin, if this has not yet been done. Additional fibers of origin from the ribs and from the inferior angle of the scapula may have to be cut to fully reflect the muscle.

86

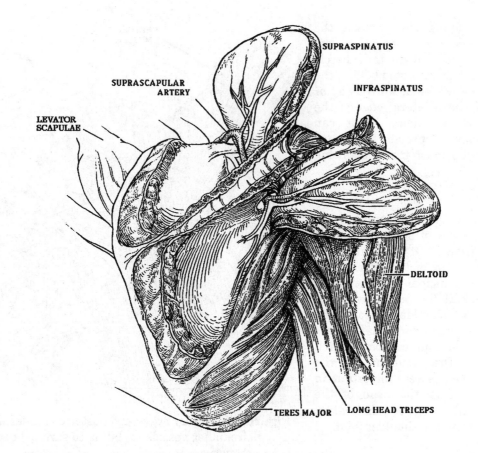

SUPRASPINATUS

INFRASPINATUS

SUPRASCAPULAR
ARTERY

LEVATOR
SCAPULAE

DELTOID

TERES MAJOR　　LONG HEAD TRICEPS

Figure 5:6 Muscles and neurovascular structures on the dorsal aspect of the scapula.

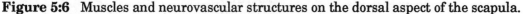

*Again identify the **serratus anterior muscle**, tracing it from its origin from the upper eight or nine ribs to its insertion upon the medial border of the scapula. Find its nerve supply again, running along the superficial surface of the muscle, near the midaxillary line; that is, the long thoracic nerve.*

The **long thoracic nerve** arises from cervical roots C5, C6 and C7 at the beginning of the brachial plexus. If the long thoracic nerve is damaged the inferior angle of the scapula flares away from the body wall, especially if the affected individual attempts to push a resistant object. This flaring is one example of scapular "winging." Because of this fact, a mnemonic poem was devised which helps one remember the nerve supply of the serratus anterior: "C5, 6 and 7 keep our wings from heaven."

In addition to the quadrangular space of the axilla, noted and dissected earlier, a second so-called "space" seen in the scapular region is of some significance anatomically and surgically. This is the **triangular space** of the axilla (Fig.

5:8). The circumflex scapular artery passes through this space, giving branches to the overlying skin of the area before turning around the lateral border of the scapula and passing deep to the infraspinatus. The circumflex scapular artery originates from the subscapular artery, one of the three branches of the third part of the axillary artery.

Deep to the infraspinatus, the circumflex scapular artery has profusely rich anastomoses with the suprascapular artery. By this means, strong collateral arterial supply can develop between the subclavian artery and the third part of the axillary artery, in the event of occlusion of the more proximal portions of the axillary artery.

*In the triangular space between the teres minor, teres major and the long head of the triceps, identify the **circumflex scapular artery**.* The circumflex scapular artery is one of the two principal branches of the subscapular artery. The subscapular artery most commonly arises from the third part of the axillary artery.

87

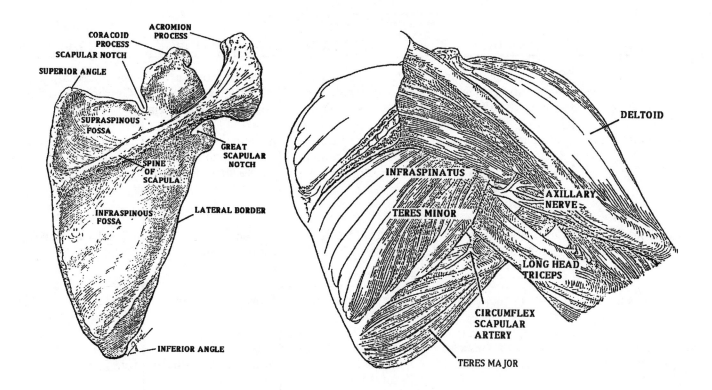

Figure 5:7 Features of the dorsal aspect of the scapula.

Figure 5:8 The triangular and quadrangular spaces of the axilla, as seen from behind. The triangular space is bounded by the teres major and minor muscles and the long head of the triceps. The quadrangular space is bounded by the same muscles, plus the humerus.

Erb-Duchenne Palsy. Many of the muscles around the shoulder receive their primary skeletal motor nerve supply from nerve fibers of the C5 spinal nerve - to a lesser degree from C6. [See Table 5:1.] These muscles include the deltoid, rhomboids, levator scapulae and the muscles of the rotator cuff. As shall be seen in the dissection of the brachial plexus, the ventral primary rami of C5 and C6 join as they emerge at the root of the neck and enter the brachial plexus.

The junction of the ventral primary rami of C5 and C6 is frequently referred to as "Erb's point." Its significance lies in the fact that so-called Erb-Duchenne palsy, or paralysis, of the upper limb occasionally occurs at birth when excessive traction upon the head results in stretch damage to the upper trunk of the brachial plexus at this point. The extent of the injury can be extremely severe, with the nerve roots torn through, or less serious trauma from tension on the nerves, with varying degrees of paralysis requiring a number of months for full recovery. With such a problem, functions of the hand are essentially normal, even though movements of the shoulder (and flexion of the elbow) are affected severely.

TABLE 5:1 MUSCLES OF THE UPPER MEMBER
- A SUMMARY -
SHOULDER REGION

MUSCLE	ORIGIN	INSERTION	ACTIONS	INNERVATION
Trapezius	Superior nuchal line; ligamentum nuchae; spines C7-T12	Lateral 1/3 clavicle; acromion process; spine of scapula	Upward rotation, elevation, retraction, depression of scapula	Spinal accessory (Cranial nerve XI)
Latissimus dorsi	Lumbar aponeurosis, spines T6-L5 (and sacrum); crest of ilium; ribs 10-12; inferior angle, scapula	Intertubercular groove of humerus	Extends, adducts, rotates arm medially; draws shoulder back	Thoracodorsal (C6, **7**, C8) (middle subscapular)
Rhomboideus major/minor	Cervical spinous processes	Vertebral border of scapula	Retract scapula, rotate scapula downward	Dorsal scapular(C**5**, C6)
Levator scapulae	Cervical transverse processes	Near superior angle of scapula	Elevates scapula	Dorsal scapular (C**5**, C6) and C3, C4
Pectoralis major	Medial half, clavicle; sternum; ribs 1-7	Crest of greater tubercle of humerus (lateral lip of bicipital groove)	Flexes, adducts, rotates arm medially	Pectoral nerves (C5, C6, **7**, 8, T1)
Pectoralis minor	Ribs 3-5	Coracoid process of scapula	Depresses, protracts scapula and rotates it downward	Medial pectoral nerve (C8, T1)
Subclavius	First rib	Inferior surface of clavicle	Depresses clavicle	Nerve to the subclavius (C**5**, 6)
Deltoid	Lateral 1/3 clavicle; acromion; spine of scapula	Deltoid tuberosity of humerus	Principal abductor of arm; flexes, extends, rotates arm medially and laterally	Axillary (C**5**, 6)
Subscapularis	Subscapular fossa	Lesser tubercle of humerus	Rotates arm medially	Upper and lower subscapular (C**5**, 6)
Supraspinatus	Supraspinous fossa	Greater tubercle of humerus	Initiates abduction of arm	Suprascapular (C**5**, C6)
Infraspinatus	Infraspinous fossa	Greater tubercle of humerus	Lateral rotator of arm	Suprascapular (C**5**, C6)
Teres minor	Axillary border of scapula	Greater tubercle of humerus	Lateral rotator of arm	Axillary (C**5**, 6)
Teres major	Inferior angle of scapula	Crest of lesser tubercle of humerus	Medial rotator; adducts, extends arm	Lower subscapular (C**5**, 6)
Serratus anterior	Ribs 1-8	Vertebral border of scapula	Protracts scapula; rotates glenoid fossa up and down	Long thoracic (C5, 6, 7)

QUESTIONS FOR REVIEW AND STUDY

1. Matching (motor supply):

a.___ teres minor
b.___ deltoid
c.___ teres major
d.___ latissimus dorsi
e.___ serratus anterior
f.___ omohyoid
g.___ levator scapulae
h.___ rhomboideus major
i.___ rhomboideus minor
j.___ supraspinatus
k.___ infraspinatus
l.___ subscapularis

A. suprascapular nerve
B. dorsal scapular nerve
C. thoracodorsal nerve
D. long thoracic nerve
E. axillary nerve
F. upper subscapular nerve
G. ansa cervicalis
H. lower subscapular nerve

a - E
b - E
c - H
d - C
e - D
f - G
g - B
h - B
i - B
j - A
k - A
l - F, H

2. What are the boundaries of :

The quadrangular space, when viewed from its posterior aspect?

Teres minor, humerus, long head of triceps, teres major

The quadrangular space, when viewed from its anterior aspect?

Subscapularis, humerus, long head of triceps, teres major.

3. What structures pass through the quadrangular space?

Axillary nerve, posterior humeral circumflex artery and veins

4. What are the boundaries of the triangular space as seen (a) anteriorly?   (b) posteriorly?

a. Subscapularis, teres major, long head of triceps
b. Teres minor, teres major, long head of triceps

5. What structures pass through the triangular space?

Circumflex scapular vessels

6. What is the origin, the termination of:
   a. the cephalic vein?
   b. the basilic vein?

a. Lateral aspect of dorsal venous arch of hand; axillary vein

b. Medial aspect of dorsal venous arch of hand; combines with brachial venae comitantes to form the axillary vein.

7. a. What muscle is the principal abductor of the arm (shoulder joint)?

a. deltoid

   b. What muscle initiates abduction?

b. supraspinatus

8. What is the origin, the insertion of the deltoid muscle?

Origin: lateral 1/3 clavicle; acromion and spine of scapula
Insertion: deltoid tuberosity

What are the actions produced by this muscle?

The deltoid is the principal abductor of the arm; it also flexes, extends, and rotates the arm medially and laterally

9. What are the origin and insertion of the subscapularis muscle?

Origin: subscapular fossa
Insertion: lesser tubercle of humerus
Function: It rotates the arm medially and adducts it.

10. What muscles form the rotator cuff?

Supraspinatus, infraspinatus, teres minor; subscapularis

11. What structure passes through the scapular notch?

The suprascapular nerve

12. What vessels pass OVER the transverse scapular ligament?

The suprascapular artery and veins

13. What is the origin of
    a. the long head of the biceps brachii?

    a. Supraglenoid tubercle

    b. the short head of the biceps brachii?

    b. Coracoid process

14. What are the insertion and the function of the pectoralis major?

Insertion: the lateral lip of the bicipital groove of the humerus
Functions: adduction, flexion and medial rotation of arm

15. What is the insertion, the function of the latissimus dorsi?

Insertion: bicipital (intertubercular) groove of humerus
Functions: extension, medial rotation, adduction of arm

16. What is the function of the teres major?

Medial rotation of arm

17. What is the function of the infraspinatus and teres minor?

Lateral rotation of arm. These and the deltoid muscle are the primary lateral rotators.

18. What is the "SIT" group of the rotator cuff? Their insertion?

Supraspinatus, infraspinatus, teres minor.
Insertion: greater tubercle of humerus.

19. What is the principal spinal nerve motor supply for the deltoid, teres minor, supraspinatus, infraspinatus, teres major, rhomboideus major, rhomboideus minor, subscapularis and levator scapulae?

C5 is, apparently, the primary source of motor supply in most individuals; C6 contributes variably in supplying these muscles, also.

20. What are the actions of the serratus anterior?

The serratus anterior acts to protract the scapula; that is, it draws it forward around the chest wall. By its insertions upon the superior and inferior angles of the scapula, it can act to rotate the scapula either upward or downward, together with other muscles.

LABORATORY IDENTIFICATION
CHECK-LIST AND SELF-TEST

The Deltoid and Scapular Regions

Osteology:

sternoclavicular joints
acromion process
clavicle
spine of the scapula
medial humeral epicondyle
lateral humeral epicondyle
olecranon

Superficial Features:

cephalic vein
basilic vein
median cubital vein
superficial perforating tributaries
deep perforating tributaries

posterior antebrachial cutaneous nerve
medial antebrachial cutaneous nerve
lateral antebrachial cutaneous nerve

Deltoid Region:

deltoid muscle
surgical neck of humerus

biceps brachii:
long head of biceps
short head of biceps

axillary nerve
posterior humeral circumflex artery
quadrangular space

upper (superior) lateral brachial cutaneous nerve

Bursae -
subdeltoid bursa
subacromial bursa

The Scapular Region:

coracobrachialis muscle
trapezius muscle
levator scapulae
rhomboideus minor
rhomboideus major

dorsal scapular nerve

omohyoid
supraspinatus
infraspinatus
teres minor
teres major

suprascapular artery and nerve
transverse scapular ligament
supraspinatus muscle
suprascapular nerve
suprascapular artery
infraspinatus muscle

rotator cuff

latissimus dorsi

serratus anterior muscle

triangular space
circumflex scapular artery

DEFINITIONS

Basilic [Gr. *basileus*, king, royalty; from Arabic *al-basilik*, the inner - a term of position]
As cephalic below, the original Arabic term for the medial vein of the upper limb was apparently misunderstood when translated into Greek.

Bursa (p. bursae) [L., a purse; from Gr. *bursa*, a skin or hide]
This term was applied to a wineskin and also to a purse. A derivative from this word is bursar, the person who is responsible for holding and dispensing the money.

Cephalic [Gr. *kephale*, head; from Arabic *al-kifal*, the outer - a term of position]
The original term from the Arabic denoted the vein on the outer side of the arm, as contrasted with the basilic vein, the vein of the inner side of the arm. There was obviously a misunderstanding of the original intent when the term was translated from Arabic into Greek.

Cubital [L. *cubitus* , elbow; from *cubo*, I lie down]
This term was derived from the Roman habit of reclining on the forearm when lying down. The word was also used as a term of measurement; the distance from the finger tips to the elbow was known as one cubit.

Humerus [Gr. *omos* , the shoulder]
The original word which we know as humerus referred to the three bones of the region, the scapula, clavicle and the humerus. In usage, the term came to be applied exclusively to the bone of the brachium.

Omohyoid [Gr. *omos*, shoulder + *uoeideis,* the hyoid]

Scapula (scapulae) [Greek origin somewhat uncertain; *spathe*, broad or flat like an oar - or from *scaptein,* to dig]
The orginal sense of the word appears to be associated with something which is wide and flat, suitable for digging; similar to the origin of the word *spade*.

CHAPTER 6

THE AXILLA AND BRACHIUM

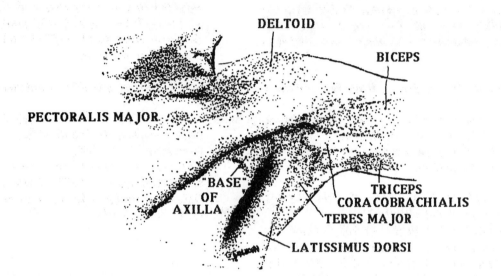

Figure 6:1 Topography of the axillary region.

Axillary Boundaries

The pectoral region should have been dissected before the study of the axilla is begun. Refer to Chapter 4 for the regional anatomy of the pectoral region and breast, if these have not yet been dissected.

In an Atlas study the structures involved in the formation of the boundaries of the axilla and then inspect this region in the cadaver. You will profit by attempting to palpate as many as possible of the individual muscular features upon yourself.

The pectoralis major, pectoralis minor, and clavipectoral fascia provide an **anterior wall** for the pyramidal-shaped axillary fossa. The **posterior wall** is composed of the latissimus dorsi, teres major, and subscapularis muscles (Fig. 6:1).

The **lateral wall** of the axilla, the narrowest boundary, is provided by a narrow strip of humerus, the short head of the biceps brachii and the coracobrachialis muscle. The upper four or five ribs, their intercostal muscles and the adjacent serratus anterior muscle constitute the **medial wall**.

The concave **base** of the pyramid is formed from the axillary fascia - deep fascia stretching between the prominent pectoral and latissimus dorsi muscles (which form the anterior and posterior axillary folds, respectively). The **apex** of the axilla is provided by the roughly-triangular, small space, the **cervico-axillary canal**, bounded by the superior border of the scapula, the first rib and the clavicle (Fig. 6:2). It is through this narrow opening that the large vessels and the brachial plexus pass to, and from the upper limb.

The Contents of the Axilla

Adipose tissue, lymph nodes and various fasciae (particularly the pectoral and clavipectoral fasciae) were noted earlier in the dissection of the pectoral region. The fascia which invests the axillary artery, axillary vein and the brachial plexus is called the **axillary sheath**. Remnants of this sheath may still remain in the cadaver, even after the previous dissections, although it is usually only poorly discerned in the embalmed cadaver. The axillary sheath is continuous with the **prevertebral fascia** at the root of the neck.

94

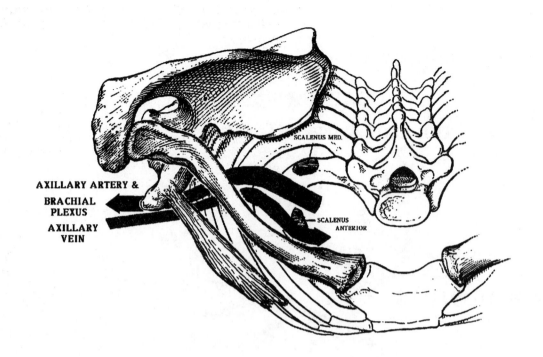

AXILLARY ARTERY &
BRACHIAL PLEXUS
AXILLARY VEIN

SCALENUS MED.

SCALENUS ANTERIOR

Figure 6:2   Course of the axillary vessels and brachial plexus. The cervicoaxillary canal, the apex of the axilla, is the area bounded by the clavicle, scapula and first rib.

Injection of an anesthetic into the axillary sheath will produce "blocking" (brachial plexus block), or anesthesia of the upper member, by its effects upon the nerves enclosed within the sheath. Numerous sites and methods of performing blocks have been described, with one of the more common being that of administration of the anesthetic into the proximal medial aspect of the brachium.

It is well to remember in this context that the phrenic nerve lies deep to the prevertebral fascia of the neck as it passes along the anterior scalene muscle. If a sufficient quantity of drug is injected, the phrenic nerve can also be anesthetized, with paralysis of the hemidiaphragm on that   side. Needless to say, bilateral brachial plexus block can cause potentially serious problems with breathing.

The anterior scalene muscle lies directly superficial to the roots of the brachial plexus just before these nerve roots pass into the axilla (Fig. 6:5)

Excise the **axillary sheath** *and adipose tissue of the axilla. Attempt to identify any* **lymph nodes** *associated with the axillary vein and its tributaries and the* **central axillary nodes** *within the fat of the central portion of the axilla.* Awareness of the positions of the principal groups of nodes is of importance in surgery for mammary disease - wherein all node bearing tissue must be meticulously removed from the axilla, to limit the spread of the disease.

Identify and clean the **axillary vein** *and* **artery**. The vein is more superficial, thinner walled and more irregular in contour than the artery. *Smaller tributaries to the axillary vein which obscure the dissecting field can be excised and removed.*

Axillary Vein. The axillary vein is formed near the base of the axilla by the confluence of **venae comitantes** of the brachial artery with the **basilic vein,** a superficial vein. [Remember: the larger arteries, such as the axillary, popliteal or femoral, are usually accompanied by a single vein.   The smaller arteries, such as the brachial, radial, tibial, etc. have two or more accompanying veins which lie on each side of the artery and are called **venae comites** or **venae comitantes.**]

Basilic Vein. The basilic vein is formed at the medial aspect of the dorsal venous arch of the hand, passes up the medial aspect of the extremity with the **medial antebrachial cutaneous nerve,** pierces the deep fascia and, with the previously mentioned venae comitantes, forms the axillary vein.   The tributaries to the axillary vein are roughly comparable to the branches of the axillary artery, but are subject to greater numbers of anomalies, or variations.

As you read the description of the basilic vein above, did you keep in mind where the "medial aspect" of the hand is, in the anatomical position? Remember also that in conventional usage the term

95

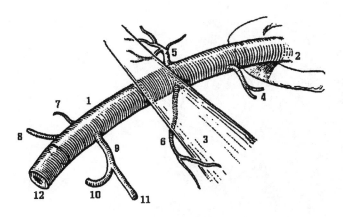

Dissection of Subclavian Artery & Vein.

The clavicles, the midline of the neck, the mandible and certain muscles are used to arbitrarily divide the neck into conveniently smaller topographic areas, the "triangles" of the neck (Fig. 6:4).

Figure 6:3 The axillary artery, 1. 2, Subclavian artery. 3, Pectoralis minor muscle. 4, Supreme thoracic a. 5, Thoracoacromial a. 6, Lateral thoracic a. 7, 8, Anterior and posterior humeral circumflex aa. 9, Subscapular a. 10, Circumflex scapular a. 11, Thoracodorsal a. 12, Brachial artery.

"tributaries to" is used with respect to veins and "branches of" is preferred when referring to arteries.

Axillary Artery. The axillary artery is divided topographically into three parts by the pectoralis minor muscle (Fig. 6:3). One vessel arises from the axillary artery proximal to the upper border of the pectoralis minor, the **supreme thoracic artery**. This small ramus provides some blood supply to the muscles of the first two intercostal spaces. Do not expend much time searching for this small artery; its presence, however, should be remembered. Do not confuse "supreme thoracic" with "supreme," or "highest intercostal artery," a branch of the costocervical trunk at the root of the neck.

From the second part of the axillary artery (deep to the pectoralis minor) arise the **thoracoacromial** and the **lateral thoracic artery**. The **anterior humeral circumflex**, **posterior humeral circumflex**, and **subscapular arteries** arise from the third part of the axillary artery; that is, distal to the pectoralis minor. *Identify each of these vessels. The veins which accompany these arteries can be removed.*

The axillary artery extends from the lateral border of the first rib to the lower border of the teres major muscle. Proximal to the first rib the artery is named the subclavian artery. Distal to the teres major the name of the vessel changes to the **brachial artery**. *The brachial artery will be studied later, but its proximal portion can be exposed now. (Note that the axillary vein becomes the subclavian vein as it crosses cephalad to the first rib).*

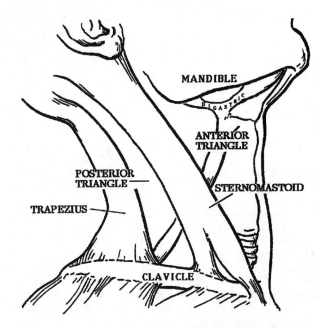

Figure 6:4 The anterior and posterior triangles of the neck.

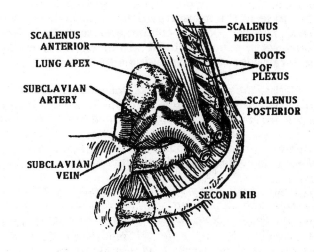

Figure 6:5 The region of the thoracic outlet.

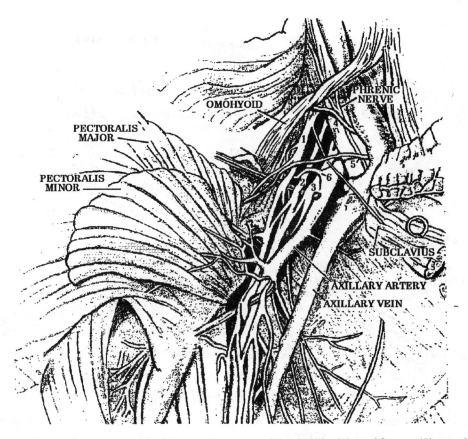

Figure 6:6 Exposure of the brachial plexus. The upper (1), middle (2) and lower (3) trunks of the brachial plexus are suspended on a probe. Note the transverse cervical (4), suprascapular (5), and dorsal scapular (6) arteries.

Two principal topographic regions of the neck are usually defined first in any discussion of the anatomy of the neck; these are the **anterior** and **posterior cervical triangles.**

The **anterior cervical triangle** is bounded anteriorly by the **midline of the neck**; the posterior boundary is provided by the anterior edge of the **sternocleidomastoid muscle** and the base is provided by the mandible. The **posterior cervical triangle** is the arbitrarily defined space bounded by the posterior border of the **sternocleidomastoid muscle,** the middle third of the **clavicle** and the anterior edge of the **trapezius muscle.**

*Reflect the skin over the sternocleidomastoid muscle and the posterior triangle of the neck. Be aware of the presence nearby of the **spinal accessory nerve** and take great care to preserve it.* The spinal accessory nerve provides motor innervation for the sternocleidomastoid and trapezius muscles.

Spinal Accessory Nerve (Cranial Nerve XI). *Incise the investing fascia which covers the sternocleidomastoid muscle from the mastoid process to the clavicle. Sever the origin of this muscle at the clavicle and manubrium of the sternum. Shell the sternocleidomastoid out of its fascial investment, leaving the fascia intact, and reflect the muscle all the way to its insertion upon the skull. As you reach the*

*vicinity of the parotid gland it may be necessary to separate the muscle from the parotid by sharp dissection. Near the insertion of the sternocleidomastoid upon the mastoid process look for, and preserve, the **spinal accessory nerve** as it enters the deep surface of the muscle.*

After supplying the sternocleidomastoid muscle, descending within it as it does so, the spinal accessory nerve crosses the posterior triangle,

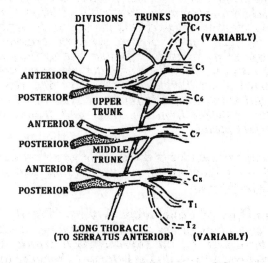

Figure 6:7 Roots, trunks and divisions of the brachial plexus

97

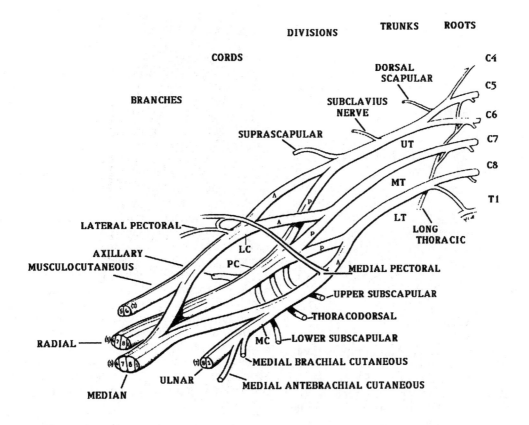

Figure 6:8 The brachial plexus. Abbreviations: UT, MT, LT - Upper, middle and lower trunks; A, P - Anterior and posterior divisions; LC, PC, MC - Lateral, posterior and medial cords.

"sandwiched" between the superficial investing fascia and the prevertebral fascia. The nerve first makes its appearance in this triangle about halfway up the posterior border of the sternocleidomastoid muscle; it then crosses the posterior triangle somewhat obliquely, passing deep to the anterior edge of the trapezius about five centimeters above the clavicle.

With a bone saw, cut away the middle two-thirds of the clavicle and note the presence of the subclavius muscle attaching to the first rib and inferior border of the clavicle. Dissect this muscle away to observe the "thoracic outlet". Reflect the sternocleidomastoid muscle to its insertion. Dissect the axillary artery and vein into the neck where the structures are now referred to as the subclavian artery and vein. Be careful not to cut the branches of these vessels or the nerve branches from the roots and trunks of the brachial plexus.

Note the passage of the subclavian artery and vein and their relationship to the anterior and middle scalene muscles.

Branches of Subclavian Artery. *Finally, clean the subclavian artery as well as possible, identifying its branches: (1) the **thyrocervical trunk**, (2) the **vertebral artery**, (3) the **internal thoracic artery**, (4), the **costocervical trunk**.*

The costocervical trunk is usually found only after some difficulty, for it arises from the deep surface of the subclavian artery. One of its branches (the highest intercostal) passes inferiorly into the thorax to supply the uppermost intercostal spaces; the other branch (the profunda cervicis) ascends in the neck, dorsal to the transverse process of the cervical vertebrae. These latter two branches need not be dissected.

*Deep to the prevertebral fascia covering the **anterior scalene** muscle identify the **phrenic nerve** (Fig. 6:6), which descends vertically upon the anterior scalene after arising from cervical ventral rami three, four and five ("keep the diaphragm alive").*

As the phrenic nerve passes inferiorly in the neck it is crossed by one or more branches of the thyrocervical trunk; that is, the **transverse cervical** and **suprascapular arteries**. *In some specimens it will be very difficult to expose some of these vessels at this stage of dissection of the cadaver. Seek advice from an instructor if necessary.*

Look for branches from the subclavian artery as it passes lateral to the anterior scalene muscle. In about 50% of people, a branch arises from the subclavian artery as the artery is crossing the first

98

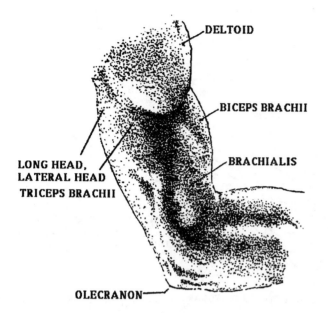

Figure 6:9 Topography of the brachium.

The Thoracic Outlet. *Review the relationships of the subclavian vessels and brachial plexus to the scalene muscles and the first rib* (Fig. 6:5, 6). The brachial plexus is a network of nerves derived from ventral (anterior) primary rami of C5-T1 and provides nerve supply to the upper member. The space between the anterior and middle scalene muscles is narrow, allowing little room for passage of the nerves of the brachial plexus and the subclavian artery (Fig. 6:6).

Several factors (cervical ribs, accessory muscles, dense fascia) can lead to compression of the neural or vascular elements, with serious consequences for the functioning of the upper limb. Spasm or hypertrophy of the scalenus anterior, the presence of an accessory scalene muscle and/or the congenital anomaly of a seventh cervical rib have been, variably, implicated in certain neural and vascular syndromes of the upper extremity. The terms applied to these problems include the "cervical rib syndrome," "scalenus anticus syndrome," and "thoracic outlet syndrome". Compression of the brachial plexus and subclavian artery between the anterior and middle scalenes can result in pain, numbness, muscular atrophy and cyanosis, ulcerations, or gangrene in the extremity - depending upon the severity of the case.

The scalene muscles, subclavian vessels and proximal features of the brachial plexus should be reviewed at this time.

rib. If this artery passes inferiorly and dorsally, deep to the levator scapulae and rhomboid muscles, it is named the **dorsal scapular artery**. Characteristically, the dorsal scapular artery passes through the brachial plexus (between the upper and middle trunks). In other people, the dorsal scapular artery is one of the branches of the transverse cervical artery.

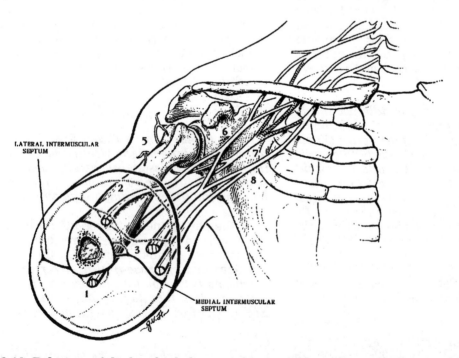

Figure 6:10 Relations of the brachial plexus and its major branches to the bones of the shoulder and the brachium. 1, Radial. 2, Musculocutaneous. 3, Median. 4, Ulnar. 5, Axillary. 6, Lateral cord. 7, Posterior cord. 8, Medial cord.

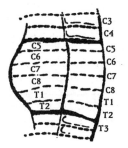

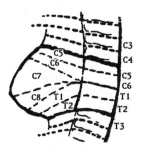

Figure 6:11 View of lateral aspect of embryo of about 30 days development, showing the early bulging of the upper limb bud and its segmental supply by spinal nerves invading from the body of the embryo.

Figure 6:12 View of lateral aspect of the embryo of about 34 days of development showing upper limb bud area. With growth of the neck and the limb, the ventral primary rami of C5-T1 are drawn out into the limb bud.

The Brachial Plexus

The brachial plexus is a network of nerves derived from ventral (anterior) primary rami. For descriptive purposes, the plexus can be divided into **roots, trunks, divisions, cords,** and **terminal nerve branches** *(Fig. 6:6-8)*. A mnemonic device you might use to remember this is, "**R**eal **T**herapists **D**rink **C**old **B**eer." [!?!]

Roots. The roots of the brachial plexus are usually derived from the ventral primary rami of C5, C6, C7, C8 and T1 ("C5" = fifth cervical nerve; "C6" = sixth cervical nerve; etc.). C4 and T2 are inconstant in contributing to the plexus. The **dorsal scapular nerve** originates from root C5 and the **long thoracic nerve** originates from roots C5-C7.

Trunks. *Re-identify the roots from C5 and C6, which combine to form the **upper trunk** (Figs. 6:5-7). Trace the **suprascapular nerve** from its origin from the upper trunk of the brachial plexus posteriorly to its passage deep to the transverse scapular ligament to enter the supraspinous fossa. This nerve innervates both the supraspinatus and the infraspinatus muscles. The large root of C7 alone forms the **middle trunk**, and the roots of C8 and T1 join to form the **lower trunk**. Each trunk splits into an anterior and a posterior division. Note these.*

The anterior divisions of the upper and middle trunks combine to form the **lateral cord**; the anterior division of the lower trunk continues as the **medial cord**. The posterior divisions of the three trunks coalesce to produce the **posterior cord** of the brachial plexus (Fig. 6:8). *Study the manner of origin of each cord on the cadaver, noting any variations.*

The cords are named with respect to their positions relative to the axillary artery while it is beneath the pectoralis minor muscle. The medial cord is situated medial to the axillary artery, the lateral cord is lateral to it and the posterior cord is deep to it.

Lateral Cord. *Identify the lateral cord and its branches, the **lateral pectoral nerve, musculocutaneous nerve** and the **lateral root of the median nerve**. The lateral pectoral nerve innervates the pectoralis major. The musculocutaneous nerve innervates the **biceps brachii, coracobrachialis** and **brachialis muscles**.

Clean and trace out the long head and short head of the biceps brachii. The short head should be exposed to its origin from the coracoid process of the scapula. The combined heads of the biceps insert by a common tendon upon the tuberosity of the radius and also by way of a strong aponeurosis which attaches to the ulna in the forearm (antebrachium). The biceps acts

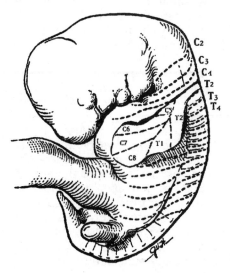

Figure 6:13 Later development of the upper limb bud at about the 40th day of embryonic development. The C6 dermatome now supplies the thumb region and the radial side of the forearm. C8 supplies the little finger region and the medial side of the palm. T1 sensory fibers are distributed to the medial side of the forearm and the distal part of the arm.

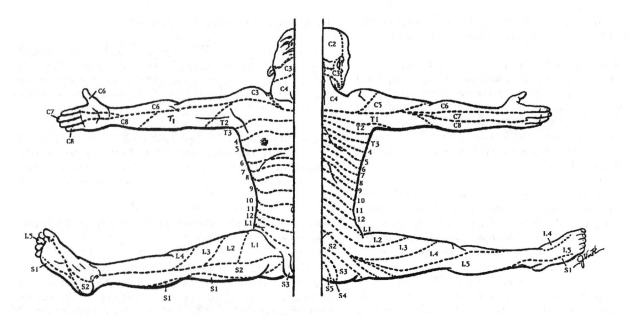

Figure 6:14 Dermatomes. C = cervical nerves 1-8,T = Thoracic nerves 1-12, L = Lumbar nerves 1-5, S = Sacral nerves 1-5,Cx = Coccygeal nerves (not shown).

The segmental distribution of the thirty-one pairs of spinal nerves to the body wall and limbs is shown in the figures above, illustrating the pattern which is present on the ventral and dorsal surfaces, respectively. Note that spinal nerves C5-T1 supply the upper limbs, and that spinal nerves L2-S2 supply the lower limbs, thus having little or no distribution in the head, neck or trunk. A dermatome represents the general region of sensory distribution of branches of a single spinal nerve. In reality, there is significant overlap of adjacent dermatomes. The above drawings represent one commonly accepted pattern of distribution; in actuality, variations in this pattern can be demonstrated clinically.

to flex the arm and forearm and to supinate the hand. The insertion will be studied in a subsequent dissection. The tendon of the long head of the biceps passes within the capsule of the shoulder joint and, thereby, also pulls the head of the humerus toward the glenoid fossa, strengthening the shoulder joint.

Trace the **musculocutaneous nerve** *deep to the biceps, to the emergence of the nerve from the lateral aspect of the brachium as the* **lateral antebrachial cutaneous nerve.**

Distally in the arm, identify the **brachialis muscle** (Fig. 6:9). The brachialis arises from the distal half of the anterior aspect of the humerus and inserts by a thick tendon upon the tuberosity and coronoid process of the ulna, to be seen later. The brachialis is innervated principally by the musculocutaneous nerve, although it usually receives a branch from the radial nerve and, occasionally, one from the median nerve.

Some reports indicate that as many as ten percent of the fibers of the brachialis are supplied by the radial nerve, so that in the event of damage to the musculocutaneoous nerve, it may still be capable of some action at the elbow joint. The brachialis is normally the most powerful flexor of the forearm (elbow joint). *Trace the* **coracobrachialis** *from its origin upon the coracoid process to its insertion upon the humerus, noting that the musculocutaneous nerve passes through the muscle.* The muscles in the flexor compartment of the brachium (coracobrachialis, biceps, brachialis) are separated from those of the extensor compartment (principally the triceps brachii) by lateral and medial **intermuscular septa.**

Medial Cord. *Identify the* **medial cord** *of the brachial plexus and its principal branches, the* **medial pectoral nerve,** *the* **ulnar nerve,** *and the* **medial root** *of the* **median nerve.** *It also gives origin to the* **medial brachial cutaneous nerve** *and the* **medial antebrachial cutaneous nerve.** *Identify and clean these branches. The median nerve should be traced to the elbow.*

The **intercostobrachial nerve** *should be noted once more at its emergence from the second intercostal space and traced out in the subcutaneous tissue of the medial side of the arm.* This nerve, the lateral cutaneous branch of T2 or T3 distributes sensory fibers to the proximal, medial aspect of the brachium and axilla. It gains some clinical interest when brachial plexus anesthesia is sought. Injection of the axillary sheath will not block this nerve, because it lies outside of the sheath and it must be infiltrated by a separate injection. Otherwise, if a tourniquet is

101

applied to the limb, the patient will experience discomfort from the compressed, sensitive nerve.

*Trace the **ulnar nerve** to the elbow, observing that it penetrates the **medial intermuscular septum** half-way down the arm, passing first into the posterior muscular compartment of the arm and then posterior to the medial epicondyle of the humerus.* Neither the median nerve nor the ulnar nerve innervates muscles in the brachium (with the minor exception noted above).

Posterior Cord. *Identify the **posterior cord** of the brachial plexus. This cord lies deep to the axillary artery and can be a little more difficult to identify and clean. There is considerable variability in the locations and ways in which its branches arise.*

*From the posterior cord arise the following branches which should be found and cleaned: the **upper subscapular nerve** (to subscapularis muscle); the **middle subscapular nerve** (also called **thoracodorsal nerve**; innervates the latissimus dorsi); the **lower subscapular nerve** (to subscapularis and teres major); the **axillary nerve** (to deltoid and teres minor muscles) and the **radial nerve** (supplies the triceps and extensor muscles of the forearm). Although the axillary and radial nerves are both quite large they are sometimes difficult to find because of obscuring connective tissue.*

*If you have cleaned the tendons of the teres major and latissimus dorsi, you will find that the **axillary nerve** and **posterior humeral circumflex artery** pass posterior to the surgical neck of the humerus just proximal to the insertion of the tendons; the radial nerve disappears posteriorly with the **profunda brachii artery**, just distal to the insertion of the tendons. Trace the radial nerve to the spiral groove of the humerus between the medial and long heads of the triceps brachii.*

The axillary artery changes its name to brachial artery as it crosses the lower border of the teres major tendon. The first branch of the brachial artery, the profunda brachii artery, passes with the radial nerve into the posterior (extensor) compartment of the arm (Fig. 6:10).

Identify the three parts of the triceps brachii. The **long head** arises from the infraglenoid tubercle of the scapula, whereas the **lateral head** and **medial head** arise from the humerus. The medial head arises from most of the posterior and medial surface of the humerus distal to the spiral groove. It is covered, hidden in part, by the long and lateral heads. The triceps muscle inserts by a common tendon upon the olecranon process of the ulna and, thereby, produces extension of the elbow joint (or extension of the forearm).

Sever the lateral head of the triceps and trace the radial nerve throughout its course in the spinal groove.

Branches of the Axillary Artery

*Review the arterial branches which arise from the first and second parts of the axillary artery. From the third part of the axillary artery, trace out the **anterior** and **posterior humeral circumflex arteries**.*

*Identify the **subscapular artery** and clean its branches, the **thoracodorsal artery** and **circumflex scapular artery** .* The circumflex scapular artery, as you will remember, can also be found within the triangular space of the axilla.

Roots and Trunks of the Brachial Plexus - Review

*In finishing this dissection, identify and trace out the **long thoracic nerve**, a motor nerve which arises from the roots of the brachial plexus. The **dorsal scapular nerve** also arises from the plexus roots and should be traced out. The suprascapular nerve and nerve to the subclavius are the two nerve branches of the upper trunk. The latter of these two nerves is usually destroyed in the removal of connective tissue as the first portions of the plexus are exposed. Review the manner of formation and the distribution of the brachial plexus.*

Neurologic Aspects of the Upper Limb. The upper limb begins as a paddle-like outgrowth from the trunk of the embryo at the levels of segments C5-T3 (Fig. 6:11, 12). Ventral primary rami of the spinal nerves of these presumptive vertebral levels migrate out into the developing limb, giving rise to the dermatomes and myotomes. A **dermatome** is, most simply, the strip of surface tissues supplied by neurons from a single spinal nerve. The dermatomes are aligned initially in a cranial-caudal distribution which later becomes more or less lateral-medial, as the limb continues to grow and undergo rotation (Fig. 6:11-14).

The normal scheme of **dermatome arrangement** in the upper limb can be remembered in a very simple schematic way:

C4: Root of neck and upper shoulder region
C5: Skin over deltoid region and lateral aspect of the arm and forearm
C6: Skin over lateral aspect of forearm and thumb
C7: Deep tissue (periosteum) of forearm and region of long finger
C8: Medial aspect of palm and little finger and the medial aspect of the distal forearm
T1: Medial aspect of elbow region and distal portion of brachium
T2: Medial aspect of brachium and axilla

T3: Axillary fossa

The neuronal process of spinal nerves grow out into the limb bud, coming to be associated with primordial muscle masses, the **myotomes**. The myotomes are arranged in a proximal-distal fashion, resulting in the innervation of proximal muscle groups by the higher spinal nerve contributants to the brachial plexus and of distal muscle masses by lower plexus contributants. This arrangement can be seen rather clearly in the following scheme:

C5: Shoulder abductors and rotators; elbow flexion (especially by biceps brachii and brachialis)

C6: Elbow flexion (especially by brachioradialis) , sensory input for biceps reflex arc; brachioradialis reflex; wrist extension

C7: Elbow extension; triceps reflex; wrist flexors; finger extensors

C8: Long finger flexors and flexor carpi ulnaris

T1: Intrinsic muscles of the hand

REMEMBER:

Motor and sensory nerves to the original embryonic flexor surface of the limb arise from the **anterior divisions** of the trunks of the brachial plexus. [Examples: musculocutaneous nerve; ulnar nerve]

Motor and sensory nerves to the original embryonic extensor surface of the limb arise from the **posterior divisions** of the trunks of the brachial plexus. [Examples: axillary nerve; radial nerve]

TABLE 6:1 MUSCLES OF THE UPPER LIMB
- A SUMMARY -
THE BRACHIUM

MUSCLE	ORIGIN	INSERTION	ACTIONS	INNERVATION
Coracobrachialis	Coracoid process of scapula	Medial surface of humerus	Flexes, adducts arm	Musculocutaneous
Biceps brachii, short head	Coracoid process of scapula	With long head	With long head	Musculocutaneous
Biceps brachii, long head	Supraglenoid tubercle of scapula	Radial tuberosity; deep antebrachial fascia	Flexes arm, forearm; supinates the hand	Musculocutaneous
Brachialis	Distal 1/2 humerus, ventrally	Tuberosity and coronoid process of ulna	Flexes forearm	Musculocutaneous
Triceps, long head	Infraglenoid tubercle of scapula	Olecranon process	Extends forearm (long head also extends, adducts arm)	Radial
Triceps, lateral head	Posterior surface of humerus, proximal	With long head		
Triceps, medial head	Posterior surface of humerus, distal	With long head		

QUESTIONS FOR REVIEW AND STUDY

1. Using an Atlas or textbook...

   (a) lightly trace the dermatones upon the following
       figures;
   (b) Identify the nerve which provides sensory
       supply to each indicated point.

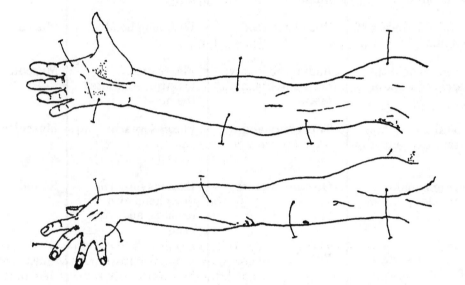

3. From what fascia is the axillary sheath derived?   Prevertebral fascia

2. Matching:

a._____	subscapularis	A. middle subscapular	a - B, C
b._____	teres major	B. lower subscapular	b - B
c._____	deltoid	C. upper subscapular	c - F
d._____	longhead of triceps	D. musculocutaneous	d - E
e._____	lateral head of triceps	E. radial	e - E
f._____	biceps brachii	F. axillary	f - D
g._____	brachialis		g - D
h._____	coracobrachialis		h - D
i._____	teres minor		i - F

4. What are the branches of the

   a. first part of axillary artery?
   b. second part of axillary artery?
   c. third part of axillary artery?

   a. Supreme thoracic
   b. Lateral thoracic, thoracoacromial
   c. Anterior and posterior humeral circumflex,
      subscapular

5. What is the manner of formation of the axillary
   vein?

   By the junction of the basilic vein with the venae
   comitantes of the brachial artery.

6. Where does the axillary artery
   (a) begin?
   (b) end?

   a. Lateral border of the first rib
   b. Distal border of the tendon of the teres major

7. What is the first branch of the brachial artery?   Profunda brachii

8. The upper trunk of the brachial plexus is formed   a. Ventral primary
   from _(a)_ rami of nerves _(b)_ and _(c)_ . Their   b. C5
   point of junction is called _(d)_ .   c. C6
                                                           d. Erb's point

9. The middle trunk of the brachial plexus is   C7
   formed from_____.

10. The lower trunk of the brachial plexus is formed   a. C8
    from _(a)_ and _(b)_ .   b. T1

11. The anterior divisions of the upper and middle   The lateral cord
    trunks combine to form _____.

12. The anterior division of the lower trunk forms   The medial cord
    the _____.

13. The posterior divisions of the three trunks   The posterior cord
    combine to form the _____.

14. The motor branches which arise from the roots of   a. Branches to prevertebral muscles
    the brachial plexus are the _(a)_ , _(b)_ , and _(c)_ .   b. Dorsal scapular nerve (C5)
                                                           c. Long thoracic nerve (C5,C6,C7)

15. The branches of the plexus which arise from the   a. Suprascapular nerve
    upper trunk (the only trunk with nerves   arising   b. Nerve to subclavius
    directly from it) trunk are the _(a)_ and the _(b)_ .

16. Name the nerves which arise from the divisions   Typically, none do. The lateral pectoral nerve, in
    of the brachial plexus.   some individuals, is formed from branches which
                                                          arise from the anterior divisions of the upper (C5, 6)
                                                          and middle (C7) trunks.

17. Each of the dots in the following diagram relates
    to a specific feature in the brachial plexus. You
    should be able to provide the proper name for each.

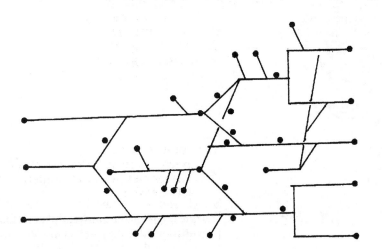

18. What spinal nerve level is associated with each
    of the following?

    A. shoulder abduction   A. C5
    B. biceps tendon jerk (motor and sensory)   B. C5 and C6
    C. brachioradialis reflex   C. C6
    D. triceps tendon jerk   D. C7

19. The following drawing depicts the axilla as
    seen from below. Identify the muscles indicated.
                                                  A. Pectoralis major
                                                  B. Biceps brachii
                                                  C. Coracobrachialis
                                                  D. Triceps brachii
                                                  E. Teres major
                                                  F. Latissimus dorsi
                                                  G. Subscapularis

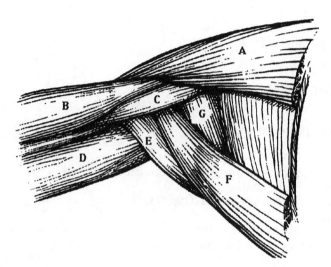

20. The following drawing depicts a parasagittal
    section of the axilla. Identify the structures
    indicated.

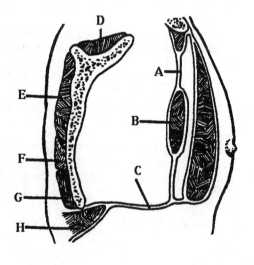

                                                  A. Clavipectoral fascia
                                                  B. Pectoralis minor
                                                  C. Axillary fascia, suspensory ligament of axilla
                                                  D. Supraspinatus
                                                  E. Infraspinatus
                                                  F. Teres minor
                                                  G. Teres major
                                                  H. Latissimus dorsi

21. Assume that the axillary artery is occluded at its
    origin. Trace an alternate route of flow which
    could bypass the occlusion.

Subclavian -- int. thoracic -- intercostal -- supreme
thoracic, thoracoacromial, lateral thoracic,
thoracodorsal -- axillary. Suprascapular--circumflex
scapular--subscapular--axillary.

22. How could blood bypass an occlusion of the axillary artery between its second and third portions?

Subclavian -- suprascapular, dorsal scapular -- scapular circumflex, lateral thoracic, etc.

23. What if the occlusion occurred between the third portion of the axillary and the beginning of the brachial?

Descending branch of posterior humeral circumflex artery -- ascending branch of profunda -- brachial artery. The only pathway, and an insufficient one.

24. Name the muscles which arise from, or insert upon, the coracoid process.

Arise from: Short head, biceps brachii, coracobrachialis. Insert upon: Pectoralis minor

25. Matching:

(1)___principal shoulder abductor	A. triceps	(1) B
(2)___initiates shoulder abduction	B. deltoid	(2) C
(3)___lateral rotation of humerus	C. supraspinatus	(3) B, D, H
(4)___medial rotation of humerus	D. infraspinatus	(4) K, F, L, G
(5)___adduction of humerus	E. biceps	(5) L, F, J
(6)___flexion at shoulder	F. latissimus dorsi	(6) B, E (long head), J, L
(7)___extension at shoulder	G. teres major	(7) B, F, A (long head)
(8)___flexion at elbow	H. teres minor	(8) E, I
(9)___supination of hand	I. brachialis	(9) E
(10)___ extension of elbow	J. coracobrachialis	(10) A
(11)___ lateral (downward) rotation of scapula	K. subscapularis	(11) M, N, O, P (upper part)
(12)___ medial (upward) rotation of scapula	L. pectoralis major	(12) O, P (lower part)
(13)___ elevation of scapula ("shrugging")	M. levator scapula	(13) M, N, O
	N. rhomboids	
	O. trapezius	
	P. serratus anterior	

26. (a) Where is the radial nerve particularly prone to injury?

a. As it passes in the spiral groove or anterior to the lateral epicondyle.

(b) How might it be frequently traumatized?

b. Fractures of humerus. Arm draped over back of bar stool; improperly fitting crutches.

27. What are the causes, and signs of scalenus anticus (Naffziger's) syndrome?

Compression of the brachial plexus and subclavian artery between a cervical rib and anterior scalene or compression by accessory or hypertrophied scalene muscles. Extra signs of the syndrome are unilateral pain, numbness, paresthesia, weakness, muscle atrophy and tenderness in the region of the brachial plexus.

28. A novice artist, painting a complex mural on the ceiling of his flat, awakens one morning to find that he cannot lift his arm (abduction) without great pain. When you lift his arm he cannot hold it in the abducted position against even mild downward pressure. Possible cause?

Possible erosion of, or irritation to, the tendon of the supraspinatus. There may also be secondary bursitis in the subacromial bursa from prolonged overhead work, with constant supraspinatus contraction (a frequent problem also of baseball pitchers). The deltoid cannot initiate abduction without supraspinatus

29. A motorcyclist, propelled over the handlebars of his bike by an encounter with a rut in the road, lands on the point of one shoulder. In addition to his injuries, his arm is rotated medially and his forearm is in the pronated position with slight flexion at the elbow.

a. What is your analysis of the probable injury?

a. Forceful downward pressure or traction at Erb's point; with tear, primarily, of root of C5, perhaps of C6 also. Tear is beyond origins of dorsal scapular and long thoracic nerves, so they are not involved. Loss of deltoid, supraspinatus, infraspinatus, teres minor muscles, biceps, brachioradialis and supinator muscles. Pronator muscles are now unopposed. Little sensory loss if C5 only is injured: if C6 is involved, some sensory loss on outer aspect of arm and forearm. Erb-Duchenne paralysis.

b. What muscles are producing the medial rotation and adduction of the arm and the elbow flexion?

b. The latissimus dorsi and the pectoral muscles produce the medial rotation and adduction. Pronators in the forearm are unopposed by the supinators. Because the forearm is pronated, muscles such as the extensors of the wrist and fingers - which arise distally from the humerus, but pass in front of the transverse axis of the elbow joint - act as weak elbow flexors. Together with other flexor muscles within the forearm, they overbalance the triceps...producing a passive flexion of the elbow joint.

LABORATORY IDENTIFICATION CHECK-LIST

Axilla and Brachium

pectoralis major, pectoralis minor
latissimus dorsi
teres major

axillary fascia (superficial and deep)
axillary lymph nodes
axillary sheath

subclavian artery, axillary artery
transverse cervical artery
dorsal scapular artery

subclavian vein, axillary vein, basilic vein

thoracoacromial artery
lateral thoracic artery
anterior humeral circumflex artery
posterior humeral circumflex artery
subscapular artery
brachial artery
venae comites of brachial artery

roots of brachial plexus (C5-T1)
trunks of brachial plexus (upper, middle, lower)
anterior and posterior divisions of trunks
lateral cord
lateral pectoral nerve
musculocutaneous nerve
lateral root of median nerve
long head of biceps brachii
short head of biceps brachii
lateral antebrachial cutaneous nerve
brachialis muscle
coracobrachialis muscle
medial cord

medial pectoral nerve
ulnar nerve
medial root of median nerve
medial brachial cutaneous nerve
medial antebrachial cutaneous nerve
medial and lateral intermuscular septa of
   brachium
posterior cord
upper subscapular nerve
middle subscapular nerve (thoracodorsal nerve)
lower subscapular nerve

subscapularis muscle

axillary nerve
radial nerve

profunda brachii artery
spiral groove of humerus
long head of triceps brachii muscle
lateral head of triceps brachii muscle
medial head of triceps brachii muscle

intercostobrachial nerve

circumflex scapular artery
thoracodorsal artery

long thoracic nerve
suprascapular nerve

suprascapular artery

DEFINITIONS

Axilla [L., armpit]
  Perhaps derived from *ala,* wing.

Scalene [Gr. *skalenos,* uneven]
  A triangle with uneven sides. The term refers to
  the form of the triangle formed by the three
  scalene muscles.

Triceps [L. *tres,* three + *caput,* head; having three
      heads]

CHAPTER 7

THE ANTEBRACHIUM

Osteology

*Palpate the **lateral** and **medial epicondyles** of the humerus, the general sites of origin of the antebrachial extensor and flexor muscles, respectively. Upon an articulated skeleton carefully study the interdependent movements of the radius and ulna as the forearm and hand are pronated and supinated. Upon yourself palpate the **styloid process of the radius**, and then the **head**, the **styloid process** and the subcutaneous portion of the **shaft of the ulna**.*

Flexor Compartment

As you study the forearm and the hand, keep in mind that, in the anatomical position, the forearm and hand are supinated (i.e., palm forward, with the thumb directed laterally). Therefore, in the following remarks, the "radial side" or "lateral aspect" are equivalent, as are "ulnar" and "medial", with respect to relative sides of the limb. Inasmuch as few cadavers exhibit hands which are fixed in the "anatomical position", descriptive information can be confusing unless you maintain proper orientation with respect to terminology.

*Prior to the removal of the deep fascia of the forearm identify the **bicipital aponeurosis (lacertus fibrosis)**.* The biceps brachii inserts principally upon the **bicipital tuberosity of the radius**. However, as the bicipital tendon enters the **cubital fossa** (the triangular depression anterior to the elbow) an aponeurotic expansion (the lacertus) arises from the tendon and blends medially with the deep fascia covering the flexor muscles, attaching then to the shaft of the ulna. These insertions of the biceps brachii contribute to its ability to flex the elbow when the forearm is supinated or pronated. In addition, because of its insertion upon the bicipital tuberosity of the radius, it is a powerful supinator of the forearm, in addition to its role in flexion.

With your hand and forearm supinated and your elbow flexed to 90 degrees, palpate the tendon of the biceps brachii as you flex the elbow isometrically (contracting the biceps brachii without actually

moving the forearm). You should feel the stout, cordlike tendon of the biceps stand out distinctly.

Now, continue to palpate your biceps tendon as you pronate the forearm and then flex the elbow with the forearm in the pronated position. You will feel the bicipital aponeurosis become taut and stand out beneath your fingertips, demonstrating its role in forearm flexion. Continue to palpate the tendons of the biceps as you return the forearm to its supinated

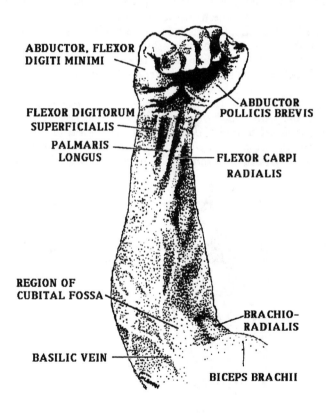

ABDUCTOR, FLEXOR DIGITI MINIMI

ABDUCTOR POLLICIS BREVIS

FLEXOR DIGITORUM SUPERFICIALIS

PALMARIS LONGUS

FLEXOR CARPI RADIALIS

REGION OF CUBITAL FOSSA

BRACHIO-RADIALIS

BASILIC VEIN

BICEPS BRACHII

Figure 7:1 Topography of the flexor surface of the supinated antebrachium.

114

position. After performing this exercise, you may be able to appreciate the European student maxim , "the biceps allows me to pull the corkscrew out of the bottle (supination) and then bring the bottle to my mouth (elbow flexion)."

The Cubital Fossa. *Remove the deep fascia of the ventral surface of the forearm, preserving the lacertus fibrosis, and then identify the boundaries of the cubital fossa.* The **medial boundary** of the fossa is the pronator teres; the **lateral boundary** is the brachioradialis (Fig. 7:1). The **base** of the triangle is an imaginary line drawn between the humeral epicondyles. The lacertus fibrosis and adjacent deep fascia form a **roof for the cubital fossa.** The **floor of the fossa** is provided by the brachialis muscle.

Reflect the bicipital aponeurosis laterally from the flexor muscles. As this is done you should be aware that this is a useful clinical landmark; this aponeurosis lies just deep to the superficial cubital veins, covering the **brachial artery** - whose pulsations can be felt at this point. The **median nerve** can also be identified here, medial to the brachial artery and its venae comitantes.

Related laterally and medially to the lacertus (or piercing it) are the **lateral** and **medial antebrachial cutaneous nerves.** What is the origin of each of these sensory nerves? The lateral antebrachial cutaneous nerve is the continuation of the musculocutaneous nerve; the medial antebrachial cutaneous nerve arises from the medial cord.

*Lateral to the tendon of the biceps, situated deeply between the brachioradialis and brachialis muscles, the **radial nerve** should be identified as it enters the forearm. It pierces the lateral intermuscular septum to pass from the extensor compartment into the flexor*

compartment. The superficial radial nerve remains deep to the brachioradialis as they pass together toward the hand. Several inches proximal to the wrist joint the superficial radial nerve emerges from beneath the tendon of the brachioradialis to begin its distribution of cutaneous branches to the radial aspect of the dorsum of the hand.

Superfical Layer of Anterior Antebrachial Muscles

Clean and separate the muscles constituting the first muscular layer of the forearm. The muscles of the superficial layer have their principal origin from the medial epicondylar region of the humerus, where they constitute a mound of muscle (spoken of clinically sometimes as the "flexor wad"). The most lateral of these muscles is the **pronator teres.** Medial to the pronator is the **flexor carpi radialis,** then the **palmaris longus** and, finally, the **flexor carpi ulnaris.**

The **pronator teres** arises by two heads; a superficial head from above the medial epicondyle, a second or deep head, from the coronoid process of the ulna (Fig. 7:2). The median nerve enters the forearm between the two heads; the ulnar artery enters beneath the deep head (Fig. 7:3). The pronator teres inserts upon the radius and, thereby, performs the function implied by its name.

The **palmaris longus** is absent in somewhat more than ten percent of subjects - either unilaterally or bilaterally. When it is present it inserts into the palmar aponeurosis, an important feature of the hand - which will be seen in the next dissection. It is useful to remember that none of the muscles of the superficial layer is involved in flexion of the fingers.

The **flexor carpi radialis** passes toward the base of the thumb and then makes its way deeply into the hand, inserting especially upon the second metacarpal bone.

The **flexor carpi ulnaris muscle** lies upon the ulnar border of the forearm, taking much of its origin from the subcutaneous border of the ulna. Distally, it inserts partially into the pisiform bone and other adjacent bones and ligamentous elements. The pisiform bone is one of the smaller bones of the wrist (carpus). You can palpate the pisiform bone as the hard little structure at the medial border of the wrist, just beyond the distal flexor crease of your wrist.

The flexor carpi ulnaris, like the pronator teres, also arises by two heads; one from the medial epicondyle, the second from the dorsal border and olecranon process of the ulna. The ulnar nerve, after passing posterior to the medial epicondyle (where it is very superficial), enters the forearm between the two heads of the flexor carpi ulnaris. The ulnar nerve innervates the flexor carpi ulnaris and the ulnar half of the flexor digitorum profundus.

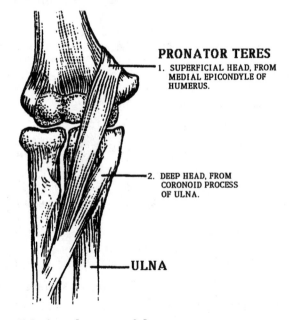

PRONATOR TERES
1. SUPERFICIAL HEAD, FROM MEDIAL EPICONDYLE OF HUMERUS.

2. DEEP HEAD, FROM CORONOID PROCESS OF ULNA.

ULNA

Figure 7:2 Attachments of the pronator teres.

The remainder of the muscles of the flexor (anterior) compartment of the forearm are innervated by the median nerve.

Trace the ulnar nerve as it passes posteriorly around the medial epicondyle, splitting the origin of the overlying flexor carpi ulnaris longitudinally as necessary to fully expose the ulnar nerve. Deep to the flexor carpi ulnaris identify and clean the **ulnar nerve and artery.** *Look for the branches of the ulnar nerve which supply the flexor carpi ulnaris and the ulnar half of the flexor digitorum profundus, the muscle which lies immediately deep to the flexor carpi ulnaris.*

In many people the ulnar nerve suffers entrapment and compression between its muscular and bony surroundings as it passes behind the medial epicondyle. The affected individual often first notes pain or a decrease in sensation along the ulnar border of the forearm and hand. In long term chronic compression, paralysis of the intrinsic muscles of the hand can also result.

Termination of the Brachial Artery. *Identify the* **brachial artery** *and its terminal branches, the* **ulnar artery** *and the* **radial artery** - the latter being usually the smaller of the two. The radial artery passes superficial to the pronator teres muscle and then, distally, is overlaid somewhat by the brachioradialis (Fig. 7:3). The ulnar artery, after giving off several important branches, passes

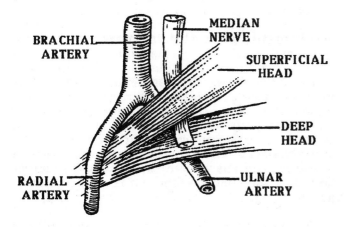

Figure 7:3 Relations of the two heads of the pronator teres to the brachial artery, ulnar artery and median nerve.

medially to lie between the flexor carpi ulnaris and the flexor digitorum profundus.

Intermediate Layer of Anterior Antebrachial Muscles

The **flexor digitorum superficialis muscle** is the sole "occupant" of the second layer of muscles of the forearm and is often considered simply as another muscle of the superficial layer. This approach to the "layering" of the muscles is especially understandable if there is not a palmaris longus muscle present.

The flexor digitorum superficialis has an extensive origin from the medial epicondyle of the humerus, the coronoid process of the ulna and from the radius. It will be seen soon that the median nerve, after passing through the pronator teres, clings to the deep surface of the flexor digitorum superficialis in its passage through the forearm.

In separating the superficial muscles you should observe the appearance distally, between the flexor carpi ulnaris and the palmaris longus, of the medial portion of the **flexor digitorum superficialis** *(sublimis). Now, divide the attachment of the flexor digitorum superficialis to the radius and reflect this muscle medially also, to expose deeper structures. Give careful attention to the relationship of the flexor digitorum superficialis to the* **median nerve.**

At the cubital fossa, again identify the median nerve and the ulnar artery. Remove any veins which obscure your view in the fossa. Note again that the ulnar artery passes deep to the pronator teres. Carefully preserving the adjacent arteries and nerves, cut the deep head of the pronator teres (if necessary) and reflect the muscle medially, so that you can trace the median nerve to its passage deep to the flexor digitorum superficialis.

Secure the median nerve and identify its **anterior interosseous nerve** *branch, which arises from the median nerve just proximal to the pronator teres. Trace the anterior interosseous nerve and its accompanying vessels deeply and distally between the muscles of the deep layer of the forearm.*

The Deep Layer of Anterior Antebrachial Muscles

Flexor Digitorum Profundus. Flexor Pollicis Longus. The flexor digitorum profundus and flexor pollicis longus arise primarily from rather extensive areas of the ulna and radius, respectively. The tendons of these muscles cross the wrist and insert distally upon the terminal phalanx of the fingers or thumb (pollux).

Pronator Quadratus. The pronator quadratus arises on the distal fourth of the ulna (flexor surface) and passes directly transversely to insert upon the adjacent face of the radius. Its function is to pronate

116

the forearm, with the assistance of the pronator teres.

*Identify and free up the **flexor digitorum profundus** and the **flexor pollicis longus**. The third muscle of the deep group can be identified distally, situated deep to the previous muscles, the **pronator quadratus**.*

Flexors of the Digits. The flexor digitorum superficialis (as will be seen in the next dissection) possesses four tendons which pass to their insertions at the bases of the middle phalanges of the medial four digits. The four tendons of the flexor digitorum profundus pass to insertion at the bases of the distal phalanx of each of the medial four digits. Those portions of the flexor digitorum profundus which give origin to tendons to the fourth and third ("ring finger") fingers are innervated by the ulnar nerve.

In most specimens, the tendon to the index finger from the flexor digitorum profundus has a nearly separate muscle belly. This is, of course, related to the considerable degree of independent movement of this digit. The flexor pollicis longus passes to the distal phalanx of the thumb. This, and the lateral two portions of the flexor digitorum profundus receive their nerve supply from the anterior interosseous branch of the median nerve.

Deep Vessels, Nerves and Muscles. As it passes deeply in the cubital fossa, the ulnar artery gives origin to anterior and posterior ulnar recurrent arteries, then to the common interosseous artery, after which the ulnar artery passes medially between the flexor carpi ulnaris and flexor digitorum profundus, where it meets the ulnar nerve.

The **common interosseous artery** is usually a fairly significant branch of the ulnar artery in the cubital fossa. It is often very short (or can be absent), giving origin almost immediately to the posterior and anterior interosseous branches. Variations in the arrangement and origins of the arteries in this area are common.

The **posterior interosseous artery** passes through, or over, the proximal end of the interosseous membrane to reach the extensor chamber of the forearm. The interosseous recurrent artery arises from the posterior interosseous artery in the extensor compartment of the forearm and ascends to anastomose with the middle collateral branch of the profunda brachii artery.

The **anterior interosseous artery** passes distally upon the interosseous membrane, between two of the muscles of the deep layer, the flexor digitorum profundus and the flexor pollicis longus. Distally, the anterior interosseous artery courses deep to the pronator quadratus. Perforating branches of the anterior interosseous artery pierce the interosseous membrane to enter, and assist in the supply of, the extensor compartment, anastomosing with branches of the posterior interosseous artery.

*Identify the **common interosseous artery**, a vessel usually of significant size - unless its two branches , the anterior and posterior interosseous arteries, arise separately from the ulnar artery, instead of from a common interosseous branch.*

*Clean the **common interosseous artery** as it passes from the ulnar artery toward the interosseous membrane between the radius and ulna. Identify the **anterior** and **posterior interosseous branches** of the common interosseous artery.*

The deep muscles of the anterior surface of the forearm are innervated by the **anterior interosseous branch of the median nerve.** *Trace out the anterior interosseous nerve again as you clean the anterior interosseous artery.*

Anastomoses About the Elbow. Proximally in the brachium, **superior** and **inferior ulnar collateral arteries** arise from the brachial artery and, with the **profunda brachii artery,** laterally, constitute the proximal portions of routes of collateral arterial supply in the event of brachial artery occlusion. The profunda brachii divides into two branches, the **radial collateral artery** and the **middle collateral artery**, which pass in front of, and behind, the elbow, respectively.

Distally, from the ulnar artery, **anterior** and **posterior ulnar recurrent** arteries arise which take part in the anastomoses about the elbow. The radial artery also gives off a branch, called the **radial recurrent artery,** near the origin of the radial artery. The **interosseous recurrent artery** arises from the posterior interosseous artery in the extensor compartment.

The superior ulnar collateral artery passes behind the medial epicondyle, together with the ulnar nerve. Because these lie on the ulnar side of the posterior aspect of the elbow, it makes sense that this artery would anastomose with the posterior ulnar recurrent artery. The inferior ulnar collateral artery descends and passes in front of the ulnar side of the elbow, where it joins the anterior ulnar recurrent artery. The radial recurrent artery passes upward, in front of the elbow, and anastomoses with the more anterior branch of the profunda brachii, the radial collateral artery.

*Identify the **radial recurrent branch of the radial artery**. It arises near the origin of the radial artery, just distal to the elbow. If you trace it proximally, you will see that it takes a path adjacent to the radial nerve. Identify as many of the other vessels of the network of anastomoses as you can, as the dissection proceeds.*

Extensor (posterior) Compartment

The extensor muscles of the hand and fingers arise from the **lateral epicondyle** of the humerus, for the most part, although the lateral supracondylar ridge of the humerus, the ligamentous tissues and the bones of the forearm also provide attachments for certain individual muscles.

Superficial Muscle Layer and Associated Structures. *Remove all remnants of deep fascia covering the extensor surface. Beginning at the radial aspect of the forearm separate, and identify, the **brachioradialis, extensor carpi radialis longus, extensor carpi radialis brevis, extensor digitorum communis, extensor digiti minimi, the extensor carpi ulnaris.** and the **anconeus**. These muscles are relatively easy to identify and separate, with some assistance from your scalpel or scissors. The **anconeus**, the most medial member of the superficial layer of musculature, is covered by a thick, tough coat of deep fascia, adjacent to the olecranon.*

The **brachioradialis muscle**, although it is innervated by the radial nerve, flexes the forearm because of its insertion upon the styloid process of the radius. It is important in flexion of the elbow, primarily when the forearm is pronated. Irrespective of its functions it is generally considered one of the extensor (or, dorsal antebrachial) muscles, because of its innervation. [Note that, irrespective of the initial appearance of the muscle as you identify it, the brachioradialis muscle does not cross the wrist joint and therefore does not participate in extension of the wrist].

*Free up the brachioradialis from its origin (lateral supracondylar ridge) to its insertion, exposing the **radial artery**, to the wrist. Also identify the **superficial branch of the radial nerve**, deep to the brachioradialis.*

After arising from the humerus, the **extensor carpi radialis longus** and **extensor carpi radialis brevis** pass distally, crossing the wrist, and insert upon the second and third metacarpal bones, respectively. The **extensor carpi ulnaris** inserts upon the fifth metacarpal bone. These three muscles are important extensors of the wrist. Just proximal to the wrist the tendons of the two radial extensors are crossed, first by the **abductor pollicis longus**, then the **extensor pollicis brevis.**

Identify and clean the extensores carpi radialis longus and brevis to the wrist. Note the abductor pollicis longus and the extensor pollicis brevis.

*Secure the **radial nerve**, proximal to the elbow. Free up the brachioradialis muscle as necessary to allow adequate exposure of the radial nerve as it divides into **superficial** and **deep branches**. The*

superficial branch passes beneath the brachioradialis, reappearing distally as it traverses to the dorsum of the hand. This nerve is sensory to approximately two-thirds of the dorsum of the hand and to the lateral three and one-half digits.

*Clean, and trace out, the **extensor digitorum** and the **extensor digiti minimi** to their disappearance beneath the tough retinacula on the dorsum of the wrist. These tendons insert upon the phalanges of the fingers.*

*Remove the tough fascia which covers the **anconeus**, so that its attachments to the humerus and ulna can be seen.* The anconeus appears to be, and functions as, a distal component of the triceps brachii muscle. It arises from the lateral epicondyle of the humerus and inserts upon the lateral aspect of the olecranon. The anconeus is innervated by a continuation of a nerve branch which supplies the medial head of the triceps brachii.

Deep Structures of the Extensor Compartment. The posterior interosseous artery passes between the radius and ulna to reach its present position within the posterior compartment of the forearm. The deep branch of the radial nerve curves from in front of the lateral epicondyle to its passage through the supinator - after which it joins the emerging posterior interosseous vessels. The **supinator muscle** arises from the lateral epicondyle and ulna and inserts obliquely upon the radius.

*Separate the superficial extensor muscles thoroughly, particularly near their origin, to facilitate deeper exposure. Free up the **extensor carpi ulnaris** from the dorsal border of the ulna to its disappearance beneath the extensor retinaculum of the wrist, and reflect the muscle to expose the site of emergence of the **posterior interosseous artery** and the **deep branch** of the **radial nerve**. Attempt to identify the **interosseous recurrent artery**.*

*With scissors, divide the planes of fibers of the **supinator** which cover the deep branch of the radial nerve. Begin this incision where the deep branch of the radial nerve first enters the supinator. Observe that the deep branch attains the posterior chamber by curving about the radius, rather than passing through the interosseous membrane as you might think at first.*

Trace the deep branch of the radial nerve and the posterior interosseous artery distally. The nerve is frequently referred to as the **posterior interosseous nerve** because of its terminal course.

*Identify and clean the **abductor pollicis longus, extensor pollicis brevis** and **extensor pollicis longus** and, finally, the **extensor indicis proprius.***

The **abductor pollicis longus** arises from the ulna and passes to the base of the first metacarpal bone. The **extensor pollicis brevis** courses from the radius to the base of the first phalanx of the thumb. The extensor pollicis longus passes from the ulna to the distal phalanx of the thumb.

Review of Motor Supply

To summarize the motor supply of muscles of the brachium and antebrachium:

(1) The musculocutaneous nerve innervates the muscles in the flexor compartment of the brachium and then terminates as a sensory nerve;

(2) the ulnar nerve supplies no muscles in the brachium, but it supplies the flexor carpi ulnaris and one-half of the flexor digitorum profundus in the antebrachium;

(3) the median nerve supplies no muscles in the brachium, but it supplies most of the muscles of the flexor compartment of the antebrachium, save the exceptions just noted; (4) the radial nerve supplies all of the muscles of the extensor compartments of the brachium and antebrachium.

TABLE 7:1 MUSCLES OF THE UPPER LIMB
- A SUMMARY -
THE ANTEBRACHIUM

MUSCLE	ORIGIN	INSERTION	ACTIONS	INNERVATION
Pronator teres	Medial epicondyle of humerus; coronoid process of ulna	Radius	Pronates hand	Median (C6)
Flexor carpi radialis	Medial epicondyle of humerus	Base of second metacarpal	Flexes hand; helps abduct wrist	Median (C7)
Palmaris longus	Medial epicondyle	Palmar aponeurosis	Flexes hand	Median (C7)
Flexor carpi ulnaris	Medial epicondyle; proximal 2/3 ulna	Pisiform, fifth metacarpal	Flexes hand; adducts hand	Ulnar (C8)
Flexor digitorum superficialis	Medial epicondyle; coronoid process; oblique line of radius	Second phalanx of digits 2-5	Flexes PIP	Median (C8)
Flexor digitorum profundus	Ulna	Distal phalanx of digits 2-5	Flexes DIP; flexes other joints with added contraction	Digits 2,3 - Median (AI*) Digits 4,5-Ulnar (C8)
Flexor pollicis longus	Radius	Distal phalanx, thumb	Flexes thumb	Median - AI (C8)
Pronator quadratus	Ulna, distal	Radius, distal	Pronates hand	Median - AI (C6)
Brachioradialis	Lateral supracondylar ridge of humerus	Styloid process of radius	Flexes forearm	Radial (C6)
Extensor carpi radialis longus	Lateral supracondylar ridge	Base of second metacarpal	Extends and abducts hand	Radial (C7)
Extensor carpi radialis brevis	Lateral epicondyle of humerus	Base of third metacarpal	Extends and abducts hand	Radial (C7)
Extensor digitorum communis	Lateral epicondyle of humerus	Second and third phalanges of digits 2-5 by way of the extensor expansions	Extends wrist, MP joints pirmarily	Deep radial (C8)

*AI = Anterior interosseous branch, median nerve

MUSCLES OF THE UPPER LIMB (continued)

MUSCLE	ORIGIN	INSERTION	ACTIONS	INNERVATION
Extensor digiti minimi	Extensor digitorum communis	Extensor expansion of fifth digit	Extends MP of fifth digit	Deep radial (C7)
Extensor carpi ulnaris	Lateral epicondyle of humerus	Base of fifth metacarpal	Extends and adducts hand	Deep radial (C7)
Anconeus	Lateral epicondyle	Olecranon	Extends elbow	Radial (C7)
Supinator	Lateral epicondyle; ulna	Radial tuberosity and oblique line	Supinates hand	Deep radial (C6)
Abductor pollicis longus	Ulna; interosseous membrane; radius	Base of first metacarpal	Abducts thumb and wrist	Deep radial (C7)
Extensor pollicis brevis	Radius; interosseous membrane	First phalanx of the thumb	Extends MP of thumb	Deep radial (C7)
Extensor pollicis longus	Ulna; interosseous membrane	Distal phalanx of thumb	Extends distal phalanx	Deep radial (C7)
Extensor indicis proprius	Ulna; interosseous membrane	Extensor expansion of 2nd digit	Extends index finger	Deep radial (C7)

Generalizations:

C_5 – Abduction and rotation of arm; elbow flexion by biceps and brachialis; biceps tendon jerk

C_6 – Brachioradialis jerk; pronators and supinator muscle of forearm; wrist extensors

C_7 – Triceps tendon jerk; extensors of elbow; finger extensors; wrist flexors

C_8 – Finger flexors

T_1 – All intrinsic hand muscles

QUESTIONS FOR REVIEW AND STUDY

THE ANTEBRACHIUM

1. Give the name of the nerve which innervates the following:

    a. pronator teres
    b. flexor digitorum superficialis
    c. palmaris longus
    d. flexor carpi ulnaris
    e. ulnar half, flexor digitorum profundus
    f. radial half, flexor digitorum profundus
    g. brachioradialis
    h. biceps brachii
    i. brachialis
    j. flexor carpi radialis
    k. extensor carpi radialis longus
    l. extensor carpi radialis brevis
    m. anconeus
    n. extensor digitorum communis
    o. extensor carpi ulnaris
    p. extensor pollicis longus
    q. extensor pollicis brevis
    r. extensor indicis proprius
    s. abductor pollicis longus

    a. Median
    b. Median
    c. Median
    d. Ulnar
    e. Ulnar
    f. Median, anterior interosseous branch
    g. Radial
    h. Musculocutaneous
    i. Musculocutaneous
    j. Median
    k. Radial
    l. Radial
    m. Radial
    n. Radial (deep radial)
    o. Deep radial
    p. Deep radial
    q. Deep radial
    r. Deep radial
    s. Deep radial

2. The biceps brachii inserts upon the __(a)__ and into the deep fascia by the __(b)__.

    a. Bicipital tuberosity
    b. Lacertus fibrosis

3. What are the boundaries of the cubital fossa?

    a. laterally
    b. medially
    c. base

    a. Brachioradialis
    b. Pronator teres
    c. Line between humeral epicondyles

4. What spinal nerve is <u>principally</u> involved in the motor supply of the...

    a. biceps brachii?
    b. wrist flexors?
    c. long flexors of the fingers?
    d. extensors of the elbow joint?
    e. flexor carpi ulnaris muscle (an exception)?
    f. wrist extensor muscles?
    g. extensors of the fingers?
    i. intrinsic muscles of the hand?
    j. brachioradialis?

    a. biceps: C5 for motor
    b. wrist flexors: C7
    c. long finger flexors: C8
    d. elbow extensors: C7
    e. flexor carpi ulnaris: C8
    f. wrist extensors: C6
    g. extensor digitorum: C7
    h. intrinsics: T1
    i. brachioradialis: C6

5. What are the insertion and the action of the brachioradialis muscle?

    Styloid process of radius; functions as an elbow flexor

6. What, in general, is the origin of most of the flexor muscles in the forearm?

    Medial epicondylar region of the humerus

7. What, in general, is the origin of most of the extensor muscles in the forearm?

    Lateral epicondylar region of the humerus

8. Identify the structures indicated in the following
    drawings:

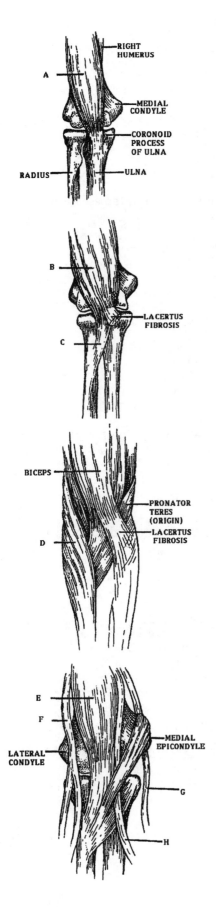

RIGHT
HUMERUS

A

MEDIAL
CONDYLE

CORONOID
PROCESS
OF ULNA

RADIUS   ULNA

B

LA CERTUS
FIBROSIS

C

BICEPS

PRONATOR
TERES
(ORIGIN)

LA CERTUS
FIBROSIS

D

E

F

LATERAL
CONDYLE

MEDIAL
EPICONDYLE

G

H

A. Brachialis
B. Biceps brachii
C. Radial insertion of biceps
D. Brachioradialis
E. Biceps brachii
F. Radial nerve
G. Ulnar nerve
H. Median nerve

123

9. What are the two principal functions of the biceps brachii?

Flexion, supination of antebrachium at the elbow

10. What muscles constitute the

    a. superficial layer of forearm?

    b. middle layer of forearm?

    c. deep layer of forearm?

a. Pronator teres; flexor carpi radialis; palmaris longus; flexor carpi ulnaris.

b. Flexor digitorum superficialis

c. Flexor digitorum profundus; flexor pollicis longus; pronator quadratus

11. What is the relationship of the median nerve to:

    a. the brachial artery?

    b. the pronator teres?

    c. the flexor digitorum superficialis?

    d. the flexor digitorum profundus?

a. Median nerve crosses the artery from lateral to medial in the brachium.

b. Passes between its two heads.

c. Is related to deep surface of muscle.

d. Lies superficial to profundus.

12. What nerve passes through...

    a. the pronator teres?
    b. the flexor carpi ulnaris?
    c. supinator?

a. median nerve
b. ulnar nerve
c. radial nerve (deep radial)

13. What muscles are innervated by the ulnar nerve in the forearm?

Flexor carpi ulnaris; ulnar half of the flexor digitorum profundus.

14. What is the innervation of all other muscles in the forearm?

Median nerve - flexor muscles
Radial nerve - extensor muscles

15. What is the innervation, point of insertion and function of the brachioradialis?

Radial nerve; styloid process of radius; flexes the elbow - most strongly when elbow is partially pronated

16. Beneath what muscle does the ulnar artery lie in the distal half of the forearm?

Flexor carpi ulnaris

17. What nerve and artery lie deep to the distal half of the brachioradialis in the forearm?

Radial artery; superficial branch of radial nerve

18. What spinal nerve supplies the dermatome of the ulnar side of the distal forearm and hand?

C8

19. What is the insertion of the...
    a. flexor carpi radialis?
    b. extensor carpi radialis longus?
    c. extensor carpi radialis brevis?
    d. extensor carpi ulnaris?
    e. abductor pollicis longus?

a. third metacarpal bone, ventrally
b. second metacarpal bone, dorsally
c. third metacarpal bone, dorsally
d. fifth metacarpal bone, dorsally
e. first metacarpal bone, radial side

20. List the arteries (shown below) which take place
    in the anastomoses about the elbow. Name the
    vessel from which each arises.

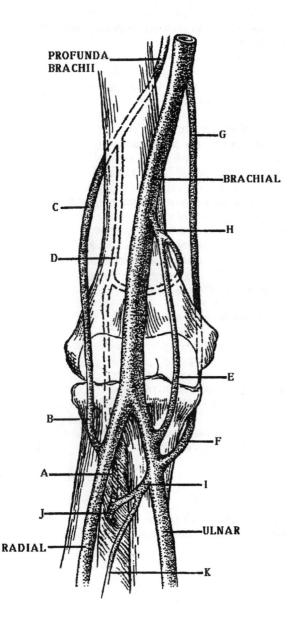

A. Interosseous recurrent - from posterior
   interosseous
B. Radial recurrent - from radial
C. Radial collateral - from profunda brachii
D. Middle collateral - from profunda brachii
E. Anterior ulnar recurrent
F. Posterior ulnar recurrent
G. Superior ulnar collateral - brachial
H. Inferior ulnar collateral - brachial
I. Common interosseous
J. Posterior interosseous
K. Anterior interosseous

LABORATORY IDENTIFICATION CHECK-LIST

The Antebrachium

Osteology:
head of radius
neck of radius
tuberosity (bicipital) of radius
interosseous border of radius
styloid process of radius

olecranon process
coronoid process

trochlear (semilunar) notch of ulna
interosseous border of ulna
head of ulna
styloid process of ulna

scaphoid (navicular) bone
lunate bone
triquetrum
pisiform bone
trapezium (greater multangular)
trapezoid (lesser multangular)
capitate
hamate bone
hook of hamate
metacarpal bones, I-V
phalanges, proximal and distal of thumb
phalanges, proximal, middle and distal of digits
  II-V

Dissection:
lacertus fibrosis (bicipital aponeurosis)
cubital fossa
pronator teres
brachioradialis
brachialis muscle

brachial artery

median nerve
venae comitantes of brachial artery
lateral antebrachial cutaneous nerve
medial antebrachial cutaneous nerve
tendon of biceps brachii
radial nerve
flexor carpi radialis
palmaris longus
flexor carpi ulnaris (two heads of origin)

superficial and deep heads of pronator teres
flexor digitorum superficialis (sublimis)
ulnar nerve
ulnar artery and venae comites
radial artery and venae comites
superficial branch of radial nerve
anterior interosseous nerve

radial recurrent artery
anterior ulnar recurrent artery
posterior ulnar recurrent artery
superior ulnar collateral artery
inferior ulnar collateral artery
interosseous recurrent artery
common interosseous artery

interosseous membrane

anterior interosseous artery
posterior interosseous artery

flexor digitorum profundus
flexor pollicis longus
pronator quadratus
anconeus muscle
extensor carpi radialis longus
extensor carpi radialis brevis
extensor digitorum communis
extensor carpi ulnaris
abductor pollicis longus
extensor pollicis brevis

deep branch of radial nerve (posterior interosseous)

supinator muscle
extensor pollicis longus
extensor indicis proprius

DEFINITIONS

Antebrachium [L. *ante-*, before + *brachium,* arm]
The part of the upper limb between the elbow and the wrist.

Capitate [L. *caput* - rounded, head-shaped]

Cubital [L. From *cubo,* I lie down - the elbow]
Pertaining to the elbow. From the Roman habit of reclining on the forearm. Cubit also was used as a standard of measurement, a distance from the tip of the long finger to the tip of elbow.

Digits [L. *digitus,* a finger or toe]

Epicondyle [Gr. *epi-,* upon + *kondylos,* condyle]
An eminence upon a bone, above its condyle.

Pronate [L. *pronatus,* to bend forward]

Scaphoid [Gr. *scaphei*, dug out + *eidos,* resembling]
Something dug out, or having a scooped-out appearance, like a small boat. The scaphoid bone has a concavity in it for articulation, which evidently led to this term for the bone.

Supinate [L. From *supinare*, to bend backward]
The placing of a person upon his back.

Triquetrum [L. *triquetus,* three cornered]

CHAPTER 8
THE HAND

Surface Features

By flexing and extending the wrist with your fingers and thumb first strongly clenched and then extended, and while moving the wrist medially and laterally, watch the "play" of the tendons beneath the skin. Attempt to identify them upon yourself and upon the hands of colleagues (Figs. 8:1, 2). After completing the dissection, you will be able to identify them with comparative ease. Upon the flexor aspect of your wrist note the distal skin crease. This crease indicates the proximal edge of the flexor retinaculum, or transverse carpal ligament.

At the ulnar end of the crease palpate the pisiform bone. By strongly flexing the wrist in a medial direction you can observe the insertion of the tendon of the flexor carpi ulnaris upon the pisiform bone. Palpate the radial and ulnar styloid processes at the lateral and medial sides of the wrist, respectively. The pulsations of the **ulnar artery** can be felt about an inch proximal to the pisiform bone, upon the radial side of the flexor carpi ulnaris.

By flexing your wrist you should be able to identify several tendons: from medial to lateral, the flexor digitorum superficialis, palmaris longus and the flexor carpi radialis. Between the tendons of the palmaris longus and the flexor carpi radialis the median nerve can be felt; indeed, pressure applied there can be quite painful. Lateral to the tendon of the flexor carpi radialis "the pulse" (of the radial artery) is usually palpated.

Removal of Skin

Make midline incisions upon the palmar and dorsal surfaces of each digit. Join these with transverse incisions at the bases of the digits; i.e., at the level of the "webs" of the fingers. With additional incisions, as necessary, reflect and remove the skin from the hand. The skin on the dorsum is very thin; that on the palmar surface is thick and tightly bound to the underlying palmar aponeurosis, from which it must be separated by sharp dissection.

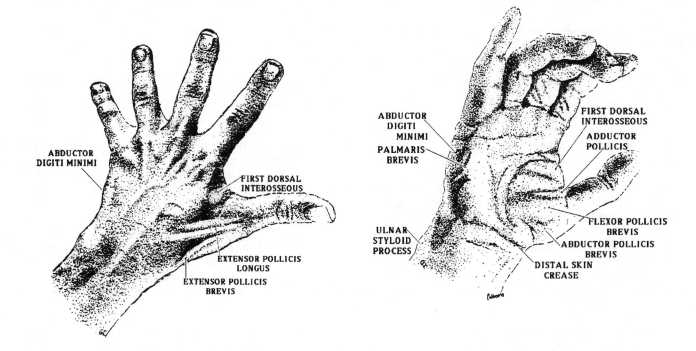

Figure 8:1 Topography of the extensor surface (dorsum) of the hand.

Figure 8:2 Topography of the flexor surface (palmar) of the hand.

Upon the dorsum of the hand identify the **dorsal venous arch;** *laterally, seek the* **superficial branch of the radial nerve;** *medially, look for the* **dorsal branch of the ulnar nerve.** *Trace out, clean and preserve them as the dissection proceeds.* The radial nerve is usually sensory to the proximal part of the dorsal surfaces of the lateral three and one-half digits and to about three fifths of the dorsum of the hand. The ulnar nerve provides sensory supply to both surfaces of the little finger, one-half of the ring finger and to the medial aspect of the hand. Although variations occur in sensory supply to the hand, it is worthy of note that sensory supply to the little finger is very consistent (and thus, clinically useful for testing the ulnar nerve).

Dissection of the Palm. At the medial aspect of the palm is the **hypothenar eminence,** which contains the muscles of the fifth digit. The most superficially placed muscle in the hypothenar eminence is the **palmaris brevis.** This thin muscle, frequently difficult to find, arises from the flexor retinaculum and palmar aponeurosis and inserts into the skin. Its contraction assists in deepening the cup of the palm. *Identify the palmaris brevis and its nerve supply from the ulnar nerve.*

Review the **flexor carpi ulnaris.** This muscle inserts primarily upon the pisiform bone, with some fibers radiating to adjacent ligaments. The ulnar vessels and nerve lie on the lateral, or radial, side of this muscle in the distal two-thirds of the forearm. Identify the **dorsal sensory branch of the ulnar nerve** which passes between the flexor carpi ulnaris and the ulna near the insertion of the muscle to attain the dorsum of the hand.

What is the innervation of the flexor carpi ulnaris? *Trace the ulnar nerve and artery into the palm, dividing the deep fascia adjacent to the lateral aspect of the pisiform bone.*

After providing origin to its dorsal sensory branch, the ulnar nerve and the ulnar artery continue into the palm lateral to the pisiform bone, superficial to the transverse carpal ligament (or, flexor retinaculum - to be described momentarily).

After crossing the flexor retinaculum, the ulnar nerve and artery give origin to **deep palmar branches,** which disappear between the abductor and flexor of the little finger. The **superficial branch of the ulnar nerve** supplies the hypothenar eminence and the palmar surfaces (sensory supply) of the fifth digit and one-half of the fourth. The **superficial ulnar artery** enters the **superficial palmar arterial arch.**

Identify the superficial and deep palmar branches of the ulnar nerve. Clean away the fascia investing the **abductor** *and* **flexor digiti minimi.** *Clean the connective tissue remaining upon the* **palmar aponeurosis.** *Trace its fibrous bands to the medial four fingers. Between these digital bands, near the*

webs of the fingers, identify the **palmar digital vessels** *and* **nerves** *and trace these out to the digits.*

Palmar Aponeurosis. The **palmar aponeurosis** contains **longitudinally oriented fibers** which are continuous from the palmaris longus, in addition to deeper, **transversely directed fibers.** The longitudinal fibers segregate distally into divergent bands which pass toward the bases of the medial four digits and assist in the formation of the sheaths of the flexor tendons. In the distal portion of your palm notice the low mounds separated by slight depressions. The depressions correspond to the positions of the digital slips of the palmar aponeurosis. Fibrosis of the palmar fascia and aponeurosis produces Dupuytren's contracture, resulting in permanent contracture of the metacarpophalangeal joints.

Divide the longitudinal bands of the palmar aponeurosis at their terminations at the bases of the digits. Carefully, protecting the digital nerves and vessels, use scissors and scalpel to reflect the bands and the palmar aponeurosis proximally toward the wrist. Reflect the palmaris longus proximally toward its origin, together with the palmar aponeurosis. The superficial palmar arterial arch lies just deep to the aponeurosis, so the reflection must be done with great care. Branches of the ulnar and median nerves will also be encountered.

Superficial Palmar Arterial Arch. *Identify and clean the* **superficial palmar arterial arch.** The superficial arch is a continuation of the **superficial branch of the ulnar artery.** Three **common palmar digital arteries** typically arise from the arch and anastomose near the webs of the fingers with the **metacarpal branches** from the **deep palmar arterial arch.**

The common palmar digital arteries then divide into **proper digital arteries,** which supply both sides of each of the medial four digits. The superficial arch is completed laterally by an anastomosis with a branch of the radial artery (either a branch of the radial artery to the index finger - **radialis indicis;** a branch to the thumb - **princeps pollicis;** or, a **superficial palmar branch** of the radial artery).

Flexor Retinaculum. *The thenar eminence contains the short muscles of the thumb. Before cleaning away the deep fascia covering these muscles reidentify the* **flexor retinaculum** *(transverse carpal ligament).*

The flexor retinaculum is a dense fibrous band that arches between the carpal bones. Laterally, it is bound to the trapezium and scaphoid bones. Medially it is attached to the pisiform bone and the hamulus of the hamate bone. The retinaculum and carpal bones form a tunnel through which the long flexor tendons and median nerve pass to reach the palm. Reduction of the size of the tunnel by disease processes results in carpal tunnel syndrome, by compression of the median nerve - with pain, paresthesias (such as burning or "tingling") or diminution in sensation from the area supplied by the median nerve, and atrophy of the thenar muscles.

Carpal tunnel syndrome is a rather common affliction, and occurs particularly in middle aged women - although its occurrence is related also to physical activity. Overuse of the long flexor muscles, for example, can result in inflammation and resultant swelling of tissues in the carpal tunnel, producing the usual signs of the syndrome. Retention of fluid due to hormonal or other factors can also precipitate the problem.

In the most common scenario of carpal tunnel syndrome, the patient is awakened in the night by discomfort in her hand. She soon finds that the signs can be alleviated by shaking the hands vigorously or by holding them under running water. Surgical correction can be achieved by dividing the flexor retinaculum, if more conservative therapy is unsuccessful.

Median Nerve. *Identify and clean the median nerve proximal to its disappearance beneath the flexor retinaculum and then, with scissors, remove the central portion of the retinaculum, avoiding the median nerve.*

Identify the recurrent branch of the median nerve. Immediately subsequent to its passage through the carpal tunnel the median nerve gives origin, from its lateral division, to a motor branch - the recurrent branch. This highly important ramus provides motor supply to the abductor pollicis brevis, opponens pollicis and the flexor pollicis brevis.

In addition to the motor supply by the recurrent branch, the median nerve supplies the first and second lumbrical muscles by motor fibers which are carried by the common digital divisions of the median nerve.

The first **common digital branch** of the median nerve provides sensory **proper digital branches** to the thumb and the radial side of the index finger. From the medial division of the median nerve arise common digital branches which supply proper digital branches to the ulnar side of the index finger, the middle finger and the radial side of the ring finger.

Thus, the median nerve is motor to five palmar muscles and sensory to the palmar surfaces of the thumb and two and one-half fingers. The distal phalanx of each of these digits is also supplied on its dorsum by the median nerve. Excepting the three thenar muscles mentioned and two lumbricales, the remainder of the intrinsic muscles of the hand are supplied by the ulnar nerve.

In most specimens a communication can usually be found between the ulnar and median nerves. Spend no time searching for it.

Review the formation and distribution of the superficial palmar arterial arch before proceeding to the deeper dissection.

Hypothenar Muscles. *Identify the abductor digiti minimi, the flexor digiti minimi and the opponens digiti minimi.* The abductor digiti minimi passes from the pisiform bone to insertion upon the ulnar side of the first phalanx of the little finger. The flexor may be difficult to separate from the abductor unless one remembers that the deep branch of the ulnar nerve passes between the two muscles near their origins, providing a helpful plane of cleavage.

Transect the abductor digiti minimi near its origin and reflect it to clearly expose the opponens digiti minimi, inserting upon the metacarpal bone of the little finger. The three hypothenar muscles are innervated by the deep branch of the ulnar nerve.

Thenar Muscles. *Identify the tendon of the abductor pollicis longus, freeing it to its insertion. Identify the abductor pollicis brevis, flexor pollicis brevis and opponens pollicis.* Note the Summary of muscle attachments at the end of the text of this chapter.

As in the case of the hypothenar muscles, the abductor and flexor brevis of the thumb can be difficult to separate. Both the abductor pollicis brevis and the superficial part of the flexor pollicis brevis insert upon the radial aspect of the base of the first phalanx of the thumb. A small, deep portion of the flexor pollicis brevis inserts, however, upon the ulnar side of the base of the first phalanx of the thumb and is sometimes called the first palmar interosseous muscle.

As stated before, the abductor brevis, flexor brevis and opponens of the thumb are innervated by the recurrent nerve. The deep portion of the flexor pollicis brevis is, however, supplied by the deep branch of the ulnar nerve.

Transect the belly of the abductor pollicis brevis, elevate it and identify the opponens pollicis. This muscle can be distinguished from other adjacent muscles by the fact that it inserts along the length of the first metacarpal bone of the thumb. (Note: it is not intended that all muscular attachments be memorized, but rather that a modicum of understanding of these is helpful, even necessary in some cases, for proper identification of muscles.)

Divide the flexor pollicis brevis near its origin, reflect it, and identify the adductor pollicis. Identify the tendon of the flexor pollicis longus. The adductor pollicis will be better seen after the reflection of the long flexor tendons to the medial four digits. The adductor pollicis inserts upon the ulnar aspect of the first phalanx of the thumb. This muscle is innervated by the ulnar nerve (deep palmar branch).

Long Flexors. *At the wrist identify the* **synovial sheath** *which encloses the tendons of the flexor digitorum superficialis (sublimis) and flexor digitorum profundus.* This sheath is named the **ulnar bursa.** The bursa extends from the distal portion of the forearm to the middle of the palm. From the latter area the sheath is continued usually only upon the tendons of the fifth digit. Digits two, three and four are provided separate mucous sheaths which begin near the neck of each metacarpal bone and extend to the insertions of the tendons (**proper digital sheaths**).

The tendon of the flexor pollicis longus is enclosed also by a synovial sheath; this is called the **radial bursa.** The radial bursa extends from the distal forearm to the insertion of the tendon at the base of the distal phalanx of the thumb. The significance of the proper digital synovial sheaths, radial bursa and ulnar bursa is: (1) that they contain lubricating synovial fluid to reduce friction; (2) that they are significant in the spread of infections from one portion of the hand to another; or even to the forearm, from the fingers or palm.

At the carpal tunnel the two most superficial tendons are the superficialis tendons to the middle and ring fingers. Those of the little finger and index finger form a deeper pair. *Free up and transect the superficialis tendons proximal to the wrist and reflect them toward the digits. Unless you have cleaned connective tissues away sufficiently in the palm and can thread the tendons beneath the superficial arterial arch it may be necessary to divide the arterial arch and reflect it to mobilize the tendons.*

Upon the fingers, incise the **fibrous tendon sheaths** *of the flexors longitudinally to trace the tendons to insertion.* These tendon sheaths extend from the distal part of each metacarpal to the distal phalanx of each digit. *Observe the* **proper digital synovial sheaths** *within the fibrous tendon sheaths.*

The fibrous flexor sheaths, like the flexor retinaculum at the wrist, prevent "bowstringing" of the tendons during the flexion of the wrist and fingers. The fibrous sheaths are thin at the interphalangeal joints (cruciate fibers) and thick over the phalanges (anular fibers).

Trace out the tendons of the **flexor digitorum superficialis** *to their insertions upon the middle phalanges of digits two through five (index, long, ring and little finger). Observe how each individual tendon of the flexor digitorum superficialis splits into two halves to allow passage of one of the tendons of the flexor digitorum profundus en route to insertion upon a distal phalanx. The individual halves spiral*

and flatten to attach to the middle phalanx, thereby forming a tendinous bed upon which the flexor digitorum profundus tendon glides.

At the wrist identify the tendons of the **flexor digitorum profundus;** *divide them, and reflect them also to their insertions. Elevate the superficial and deep tendons gently and identify the underlying, slender and delicate* **vinculi longa and vinculi breva.** Within the fibrous flexor sheath of each finger the tendons of the flexor digitorum superficialis and flexor digitorum profundus are enclosed within a common synovial sheath with parietal and visceral layers. Blood to the tendons is supplied by small vessels which pass from the ventral surface of the phalanges to the tendons, enclosed by synovial folds called **vinculi.**

A short vinculum is given off to each tendon very close to its respective insertion. A long vinculum is provided for each tendon more proximally - usually at the level of the phalanx proximal to tendinous insertion. Only the long vinculi normally carry the blood vessels; the short vinculi act as tethers for the tendons near their insertions.

Identify the **four lumbrical muscles,** *slender muscles which arise from the tendons of the flexor digitorum profundus.* The lumbrical tendons pass to the radial side of each of the medial four digits and insert into the **extensor expansion** (to be considered later) of each digit. Lumbricales one and two (to the index and middle fingers) are innervated by the median nerve. Lumbricales three and four (to the ring and little fingers) are innervated by the deep branch of the ulnar nerve.

Palmar Fascial Spaces. The palmar fascial spaces (or clefts) are actually potential spaces (Fig. 8:3) which, like the above described sheaths and bursae, are very important clinically in the spread of infection. Two of these spaces are exposed when you

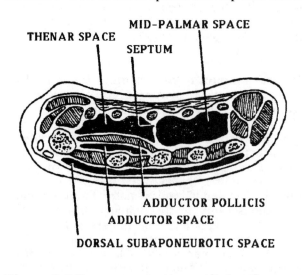

THENAR SPACE · MID-PALMAR SPACE · SEPTUM · ADDUCTOR POLLICIS · ADDUCTOR SPACE · DORSAL SUBAPONEUROTIC SPACE

Figure 8:3 Transverse section outlining the compartments of the hand.

131

reflect the long flexor tendons with their synovial investment. These potential spaces lie between the flexor tendons anteriorly, and the adductor pollicis, interosseous muscles and metacarpal bones, posteriorly.

Deep to the flexor tendons, the deep space of the palm is divided into a **thenar space** and a **mid-palmar space** by a fibrous septum which extends between the flexor tendons of the middle finger and the third metacarpal bone. The third potential fascial cleft is situated deep to the adductor pollicis and is therefore named the **adductor space** (Fig. 8:3).

Deep Palmar Dissection. *Reflect the tendon of the flexor pollicis longus toward its insertion and define the borders of the **adductor pollicis**.* This latter muscle possesses a proximal, **oblique head** and a distal, **transverse head**. The adductor pollicis arises from the third metacarpal and inserts upon the ulnar aspect of the first phalanx of the thumb (Fig. 8:4).

*Identify the **deep palmar arterial arch**.* The radial artery enters the palm by first turning dorsally at the wrist, and then passes between the two heads of the first dorsal interosseous muscle. Thereafter it passes into the deep aspect of the palm between the oblique and transverse heads of the adductor pollicis. The deep arterial arch is completed by an anastomosis of the radial artery with the **deep branch of the ulnar artery.**

*Trace the **deep branch of the ulnar nerve** into the palm by dividing the origins of the short muscles of the little finger as necessary.*

The deep branch of the ulnar nerve innervates the three hypothenar muscles, two lumbricales, all of the interossei muscles and the adductor pollicis. The nerve passes deep to the fascial clefts, accompanied by the deep palmar arterial arch to its passage into the adductor pollicis. There, it supplies the adductor pollicis and the deep head of the flexor pollicis brevis.

With scissors, divide the origin of the adductor pollicis and reflect it toward its insertion to better expose the course of the radial artery.

The Interossei. The **midline of the hand** is considered to be a line drawn longitudinally through the middle finger. The dorsal and palmar interossei abduct and adduct, respectively, the medial four digits away from or toward this line. There are four dorsal and three palmar interosseous muscles (Fig. 8:4).

The first dorsal interosseous muscle inserts upon the **radial** side of the index finger; the second and third dorsal interossei insert upon **either** side of the middle finger; the fourth dorsal interosseous muscle inserts upon the **ulnar** side of the ring finger.

Because of these attachments the dorsal interossei **abduct** the index, middle and ring fingers from the midline of the hand.

The first palmar interosseous muscle inserts upon the **ulnar** side of the index finger; the second palmar interosseous muscle inserts upon the **radial** side of the ring finger; the third palmar interosseous muscle inserts upon the **radial** side of the little finger. The palmar interossei therefore **adduct** the index, ring and little fingers toward the midline of the hand.

*Identify the **first dorsal** and **first palmar interosseous muscles**.* The first dorsal interosseous muscle is seen best from a dorsal view of the hand. It arises from the first and second metacarpal bones. Between these two heads of origin the radial artery passes into the palm, emerging in the deep palm between the two heads of the adductor pollicis.

The interossei, both dorsal and palmar (volar), insert partially upon the base of the first phalanx of each of the medial four digits; but, like the lumbricales, they insert also into the extensor expansions of the digits.

Because of the insertion of the lumbricales and interossei into the extensor expansions, they not only abduct and adduct, but **they flex the metacarpophalangeal joints and extend the interphalangeal joints of the fingers.**

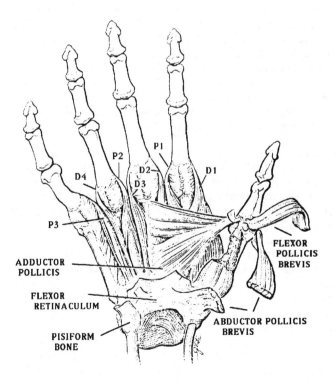

Figure 8:4 Deep dissection of the hand showing some of the deep intrinsic muscles. P1-P3, palmar interossei. D1-D4, dorsal interossei.

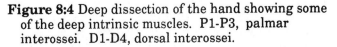

Extensor Aspect of the Hand

Upon the dorsum of the hand, divide and remove the fascia and extensor retinaculum from the tendons crossing the wrist, tracing each tendon to its insertion.

Trace the **extensor pollicis brevis** *to the base of the first phalanx, and the* **extensor pollicis longus** *to the base of the distal phalanx of the thumb.* The tendons of these two muscles form the boundaries of the **"anatomical snuff-box,"** through which the radial artery passes to reach the dorsum of the thumb. *Observe the following characteristics of the anatomical snuffbox:*

The **floor** of the snuffbox is formed by the radial artery, lying upon the scaphoid bone.

The **roof** of the snuffbox contains the cephalic vein and the superficial branch of the radial nerve.

The **lateral wall** of the snuffbox contains the tendons of the abductor pollicis longus and the extensor pollicis brevis.

The **medial wall** of the snuffbox is provided by the tendon of the extensor pollicis longus.

If you have not already done so, expose the radial artery on the dorsum of the base of the thumb and trace it to its disappearance through the two heads of the first dorsal interosseous muscle.

Trace the tendons of the **extensor carpi radialis longus** *and* **brevis** *to their insertions.*

Demonstrate the tendons of the **extensor digitorum communis**, *noting: (1) the* **tendinous interconnections** *between the tendons to the medial three fingers; (2)* **expansions,** *or "hoods" from the extensor tendons at the base of each finger, distal to its metacarpal. Identify, clean and trace the tendons of insertion of the lumbricales and interossei into the extensor expansion of either the third or fourth finger.*

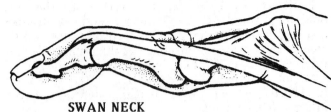

SWAN NECK

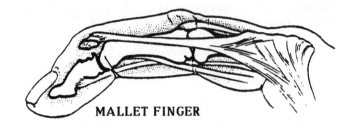

MALLET FINGER

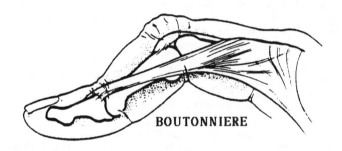

BOUTONNIERE

Figure 8:5 Disorders of the extensor expansion of the digits.

133

Each extensor hood has an insertion into the first phalanx of the digit. The extensor tendon continues distally, supplemented by **lateral bands** which receive the tendons of insertion of the lumbricals and interossei. It is by their insertions into this dorsal extensor mechanism that the interossei and lumbricals act as the principal extensors of the interphalangeal joint.

The extensor mechanisms of the digits are extremely important in the functions of the fingers. Injuries to them are not uncommon, including the so-called "swan neck," "mallet finger" and "boutonniere" deformities (Fig. 8:5) - which are further described in the Questions section.

TABLE 8:1 MUSCLES OF THE UPPER LIMB
- A SUMMARY -
THE HAND

MUSCLE	ORIGIN	INSERTION	ACTIONS	INNERVATION
Abductor pollicis brevis	Flexor retinaculum; scaphoid, trapezium	Radial side, base of first phalanx, thumb	Abducts thumb	Median - recurrent
Opponens pollicis	Flexor retinaculum and trapezium	Radial side, first metacarpal	Abducts, flexes and rotates thumb	Median - recurrent
Flexor pollicis brevis	Supf. - flexor retinaculum and trapezium Deep - first metacarpal	Radial side, first phalanx Ulnar side, first phalanx	Flexes and adducts thumb	Median - recurrent Ulnar - deep branch
Adductor pollicis	Transverse head: third metacarpal Oblique head: bases of 2nd and 3rd metacarpals	Ulnar side, first phalanx of thumb	Adducts thumb	Ulnar - deep branch
Palmaris brevis	Transverse carpal ligament; palmar aponeurosis	Skin of palm	Deepens palm	Ulnar
Abductor digiti minimi	Pisiform bone	Ulnar side, first phalanx of fifth digit	Abducts and flexes first phalanx	Ulnar - deep branch
Flexor digiti minimi	Hamate hamulus; flexor retinaculum	Flexor surface of first phalanx, fifth digit	Adducts, flexes and rotates 5th digit	Ulnar - deep branch
Opponens digiti Minimi	Hamate hamulus	Fifth metacarpal, ulnar side	Abducts and flexes 5th digit	Ulnar - deep branch
Lumbricales	Tendons of flexor digitorum profundus	Extensor expansion of digits 2-5, radial side	Flex MP; extend PIP, DIP	Med. to 1 & 2 Ulnar to 3 & 4
Palmar Interossei	Each arises from the side of one metacarpal	Into base of first phalanx and ext. expansion of same digit as origin	Adduct 2nd, 4th, and 5th digits; flex MP and extend IP joints	Ulnar - deep branch
Dorsal Interossei	Each arises from adjacent sides of two metacarpals	Into base of first phalanx and ext. expansion of 2nd, 3rd, and 4th digits.	Abduct 2nd, 3rd, 4th digits; flex MP and extend IP joints	Ulnar - deep branch

QUESTIONS FOR REVIEW AND STUDY

1. What is the innervation of:

   a. abductor digiti minimi   a. Deep branch, ulnar
   b. flexor digiti minimi   b. Deep branch, ulnar
   c. opponens digiti minimi   c. Deep branch, ulnar
   d. palmaris brevis   d. Ulnar nerve
   e. lumbricales III, IV   e. Deep branch, ulnar
   f. dorsal and palmar interossei   f. Deep branch, ulnar
   g. adductor pollicis   g. Deep branch, ulnar
   h. abductor pollicis brevis   h. Recurrent branch, median
   i. flexor pollicis brevis   i. Recurrent branch, median
   j. opponens pollicis   j. Recurrent branch, median
   k. lumbricales I, II   k. Median nerve
   l. abductor pollicis longus   l. Deep branch, radial
   m. extensor pollicis longus   m. Deep branch, radial
   n. extensor pollicis brevis   n. Deep branch, radial
   o. extensor digitorum communis   o. Deep branch, radial
   p. flexor digitorum superficialis   p. Median
   q. flexor digitorum profundus, medial one-half   q. Ulnar nerve
   r. flexor digitorum profundus, lateral one-half   r. Anterior interosseous, median
   s. flexor pollicis longus   s. Anterior interosseous, median

2. Sensory supply of the hand:

   a.____Medial border, little finger, one-half ring finger   a. Ulnar
   b.____Lateral aspect of dorsum of hand   b. Radial
   c.____Palmar surfaces of lateral three and one-half digits   c. Median

3. What are the boundaries of the "anatomical snuff-box" or tabatiere? What vessels are situated in this area?

   Radial side: tendons of extensor pollicis brevis and abductor pollicis longus
   Ulnar side: tendon of extensor pollicis longus
   Superficial: cephalic vein (with superficial radial nerve);
   Deep: radial artery

4. Name the structures that pass through the carpal tunnel.

   Tendons of flexor digitorum superficialis, profundus and pollicis longus; median nerve

5. The radial artery, ulnar artery and ulnar nerve pass _____to the flexor retinaculum.

   Superficial

6. The main contributant to the superficial palmar arterial arch is the __(a)__artery, that to the deep arch is from the __(b)__artery.

   a. Ulnar
   b. Radial

7. What is the insertion of the:
   a. flexor digitorum profundus?   a. base of distal phalanx
   b. flexor digitorum superficialis?   b. base of middle phalanx
   c. lumbricales?   c. extensor expansion
   d. interossei?   d. extensor expansion, first phalanx
   e. opponens pollicis?   e. metacarpal of thumb

8. What are the functions of the palmar interossei?

Adduction of digits II, IV and V; flex MP joints, and extend IP joints

9. What are the functions of the dorsal interossei?

Abduction of digits II, III, and IV; flex MP joints, extends IP joints

10. What are the functions of the lumbricales?

Flex MP joints, extend IP joints

11. The ulnar nerve and artery pass _____ to the palmar carpal ligament.

Deep....Note that the palmar carpal ligament is proximal to, and superficial to, the flexor retinaculum (transverse carpal ligament).

12. Matching:

a.___first lumbrical	A. Median	a. A
b.___2nd lumbrical	B. Ulnar	b. A
c.___3rd lumbrical	C. Radial	c. B
d.___4th lumbrical	D. None of the above	d. B
e.___dorsal interossei		e. B
f.___palmar interossei		f. B
g.___adductor pollicis longus		g. B
h.___flexor pollicis longus		h. A
i.___flexor pollicis longus		i. A
j.___abductor pollicis longus		j. C
k.___abductor pollicis brevis		k. A
l.___extensor pollicis longus		l. C
m.___flexor digitorum sublimis		m. A
n.___flexor digitorum profundus, medial 1/2		n. B
o.___opponens digiti minimi		o. B
p.___flexor digiti minimi		p. B
q.___opponens pollicis		q. A
r.___palmaris brevis		r. B
s.___extensor indicis proprius		s. C
t.___abductor digiti minimi		t. B
u.___sensory, surface of fifth and one-half fourth digit		u. B
v.___sensory, palmar surface of three and one-half digits		v. A
w.___sensory, dorsal surface of three and one-half digits (proximally)		w. C

13. The accompanying drawing depicts a cross section of the wrist. Identify the tendons in each compartment.

Compartment and Contents

IA	abductor pollicis longus
IB	extensor pollicis brevis
IIA	extensor carpi radialis longus
IIB	extensor carpi radialis brevis
III	extensor pollicis longus
IVA	extensor digitorum communis
IVB	extensor indicis
V	extensor digiti minimi
VI	extensor carpi ulnaris

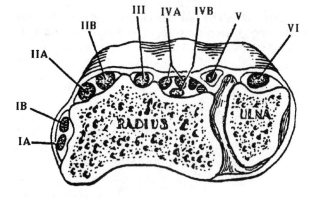

14. The _____ligament is the distal portion of the investing antebrachial fascia which is especially thickened at the wrist.

Palmar, or volar carpal ligament

15. Use the diagram below to answer the following questions. The __(A)__ligament is a thick fibrous band   which forms a tunnel beneath which the long   flexor tendons and median nerve pass. It is attached medially to the __(B)__and _____ bones and laterally to the __(C)_____ and_____.

A. Transverse carpal ligament (flexor retinaculum)
B. Pisiform and hook of hamate
C. Scaphoid and trapezium

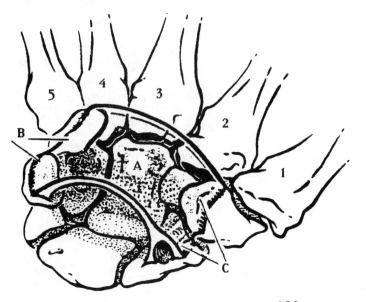

16. Name each deformity and explain its causes:

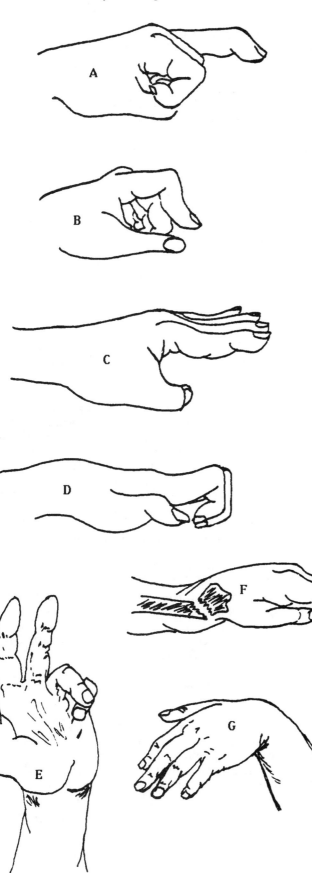

A. Mallet finger: Caused by rupture of DIP (distal interphalangeal) extensor mechanism or avulsion fracture of dorsal portion of distal phalanx. Common in baseball catchers. Flexor profundus pulls DIP into flexion. Cannot extend DIP.

B. Boutonniere deformity: Central portion of extensor expansion torn over the PIP (proximal interphalangeal) joint; allows tendon to fall palmward and become a PIP flexor and by shortening, to cause DIP hyperextension; thus PIP flexed, DIP hyperextended.

C. Swan-neck deformity of fingers: flexion of MP, PIP hyperextension, slight DIP flexion; due to shortening or contracture of intrinsic muscles and tendons, as in rheumatoid arthritis.

D. Claw-hand deformity. The figure illustrates the clawing which follows injury to both the median and the ulnar nerves. With ulnar loss alone, the defect is seen in the 4th and 5th digits, primarily; less in digits 2 and 3, because the first two lumbricales are still innervated (median), lessening the clawing. Intact long extensors cause extension of the MP joints (hyperextension, usually); PIP and DIP joints kept flexed by intact long and short finger flexors.

E. Dupuytren's contracture: Flexion contracture of the fourth and fifth digits, due to fibrosis of palmar fascia (not flexor tendons); mostly associated with aging, beginning as fibrous nodules which progress to dense contraction bands.

F. Dinner fork deformity: Colles' fracture of the wrist; fracture of distal inch of radius causing dorsal angulation of distal fragment.

G. Wrist drop deformity: radial nerve paralysis produces inability to extend MP joints, although PIP and DIP can be extended by the intact median and ulnar innervated muscles.

17. The anterior tibial artery is to the interosseous membrane of the leg as the __(a)__ artery is to the interosseous membrane of the forearm. The common peroneal nerve is comparable in its course about the __(b)__ as the __(c)__ nerve in its course about the radius.

a. posterior interosseous artery
b. fibula
c. deep branch of radial nerve

18. With what structure in the upper member is each of the following comparable?

a. femur
b. flexor hallucis longus
c. medial plantar nerve
d. great saphenous vein
e. short saphenous vein
f. quadriceps femoris muscle
g. rectus femoris muscle
h. lateral plantar nerve

a. humerus
b. flexor pollicis longus
c. median nerve in hand
d. cephalic vein
e. basilic vein
f. triceps brachii muscle
g. long head of triceps brachii
h. ulnar nerve in the hand

19. What is the most frequent injury to the carpal bones? What is the characteristic clinical sign of it?

Fall upon the hand with fracture of the scaphoid bone; tenderness and swelling over the anatomical snuff-box results. Ischemic necrosis of bone fragments can increase the severity of the injury.

20. What may be the cause of pain, paresthesias - with weakness, paralysis, or atrophy of the thenar muscles, with no external indication of injury?

Carpal tunnel syndrome (median nerve neuritis at the wrist); results from any derangement which reduces the diameter of the carpal tunnel or increases the pressure within it - resulting in compression of the median nerve. Most frequently occurs in middle-aged women, but also see in laborers and truck drivers.

21. What is the "million-dollar" nerve? How can it be located?

The recurrent branch of the median nerve, which innervates three important intrinsic muscles of the thumb. Touch the tip of the ring finger to the base of the thenar eminence.

22. What is the "retrotendinous space of Parona?"

A clinical term used to describe the continuity of the space behind the flexor pollicis longus and flexor digitorum profundus tendons with the deep palmar spaces. Infections and toxins can spread from the palm into the forearm by this route.

23. How does the radial artery enter the palm?

By passing between the two heads of the first dorsal interosseous muscle.

24. a. Where do the palmar metacarpal arteries arise?
    b. The proper digital arteries?

a. From the deep palmar arterial arch. They anastomose with the common digital branches of the superficial arch.
b. The proper digital arteries arise from the common digital arteries, distal to this anastomosis.

141

25. Identify the sources of sensory supply to the
hand.

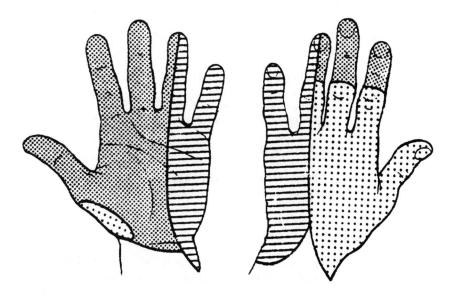

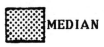MEDIAN

ULNAR

RADIAL

LABORATORY IDENTIFICATION CHECK-LIST

The Hand

flexor retinaculum (transverse carpal ligament)
pisiform bone
tendon of flexor carpi ulnaris
ulnar artery

flexor digitorum superficialis (sublimis)
palmaris longus
flexor carpi radialis
median nerve

dorsal venous arch
superficial branch of radial nerve
dorsal branch of ulnar nerve

hypothenar eminence
palmaris brevis

flexor carpi ulnaris

deep palmar branches of ulnar artery and nerve
superficial branch of ulnar nerve
superficial ulnar artery

abductor digiti minimi
flexor digiti minimi

palmar aponeurosis - digital slips
transverse and longitudinal fibers of aponeurosis

superficial palmar arterial arch
common palmar digital arteries
proper digital arteries
thenar eminence

flexor retinaculum

median nerve
recurrent branch of median nerve
common digital branches of median nerve
proper digital branches of median nerve

abductor digiti minimi
flexor digiti minimi brevis
opponens digiti minimi

abductor pollicis brevis
flexor pollicis brevis
opponens pollicis
tendon of flexor pollicis longus

ulnar bursa

fibrous flexor tendon sheaths
proper digital synovial sheath

vinculi longa
vinculi breva

lumbrical muscles, digits II - V
nerves to lumbricals (first and second)

radial bursa
adductor pollicis (oblique and transverse heads)
deep palmar arterial arch

radial artery in palm
radialis indicis artery
princeps pollicis artery
superficial palmar branch of radial artery
deep branch of ulnar artery

branches of deep ulnar nerve
first dorsal interosseous muscle
dorsal and palmar interossei
extensor pollicis brevis
extensor pollicis longus
anatomical snuff-box
extensor expansions
tendinous interconnections (juncturae tendinum)

DEFINITIONS

Hypothenar [Gr. *hypo-,* under + *thenar,* palm]
The fleshy eminence on the ulnar side of the palm.

Lumbrical (pl. lumbricales or lumbricals) [L. *lumbricus,* a worm]
Small, worm-shaped muscles which arise from the deep flexor tendons in the hands and feet.

Retinaculum (pl. retinacula) [L. "a rope, cable"]
A structure which retains an organ or tissue in place.

Vinculum (pl. vincula) [L. From *vincio,* to bind; a fetter]

CHAPTER 9

THE ARTICULATIONS OF THE UPPER MEMBER

Inasmuch as relatively little time is required for this initial dissection of the joints of the upper limb one may also be inclined to casually dismiss study of them as being of little interest. The therapist, however, knows that joint separations, dislocations and dysfunction due to disease are of common occurrence and are not lightly regarded by the ones who must endure them. Therefore, the details of their structure and their clinical relevance are considerably greater than indicated here.

General Considerations

Joints can be divided into three major classes: **immovable** (synarthroses; e.g., sutural joints of the skull), **partially movable** (amphiarthroses; e.g., intervertebral disks, symphysis pubis) and **freely movable** (diarthroses, the majority of joints).

The freely movable joints include the hinge, pivot, ball-and-socket, gliding, elipsoidal (condyloid) and the saddle type of joint. Irrespective of their form and function each of these joint types possesses the first four, or all, of the following characteristics:
(1) **hyaline cartilage** on the articular surfaces of the bones;
(2) a **fibrous capsule** which joins the articulating surfaces of the bones involved in the joint;
(3) a **synovial membrane** within the joint capsule, which produces the lubricating synovial fluid;
(4) **ligaments** which join the articulating bones and add strength to the joint;
(5) a synovial membrane-covered **articular disk** which intervenes between adjacent bones.

The ligaments associated with a joint may be heavy, cordlike, and distinct, or be merely thickenings of portions of the fibrous capsule. In some joints the most significant factor providing strength and stability is neither the fibrous capsule nor the associated ligaments, but rather **muscles** and/or tendons which pass about, or cover the joint.

Hilton's Law. Neural supply to a joint is usually provided by rami from the nerves which innervate the muscles which act upon the joint.

The joints to be studied in this dissection include: (1) a metacarpophalangeal joint; (2) the carpometacarpal joint of the thumb; (3) the wrist; (4) the elbow; (5) attachments of the pectoral girdle; (6) the shoulder joint.

Joints of the Hand

Metacarpophalangeal Joints. The articulations of the metacarpal bones with the proximal phalanges are strengthened by fibrocartilaginous palmar plates; the tendons which cross the joints; the fibrous capsule, and the collateral ligaments (Fig. 9:1).

The **metacarpophalangeal (MP) joints** are of the **elipsoidal** type; that is, formed by the juxtaposition of the rounded head of the metacarpal bones and the shallow depressions of the proximal ends of the phalanges. Such joints permit flexion, extension, abduction, adduction and circumduction. What is the difference between circumduction and rotation?

*Remove the soft tissues and extensor apparatus from the dorsum and sides of one MP joint to expose the **fibrous articular capsule**. With scissors, trim away a small portion of the capsule on the dorsal aspect of the joint. Identify the two **collateral ligaments**, one on either side of the joint. Note that these ligaments are **relaxed** when the digit is **extended, taut** when **flexed** because of (1) the obliquity of the ligaments, passing from the dorsal aspect of the metacarpal bone to the palmar surface of the phalanx; (2) the curvatures of the head of the metacarpal bone.*

Attempt to abduct and adduct your fingers when they are extended; partially flexed; fully flexed. What differences do you observe? The **proximal interphalangeal joints** ("PIP" joints) and **distal interphalangeal joints** ("DIP" joints) also possess collateral ligaments, but need not be dissected. These are simple hinge-type (ginglymus) joints.

Carpo-Metacarpal Joint of Thumb. The carpometacarpal joint of the thumb principally involves the articulation of the **trapezium** bone with the **first metacarpal** bone. This joint exemplifies the "**saddle-type**" **joint** and can be flexed, extended, abducted, adducted and circumducted, and is capable even of a slight degree of rotation. Which of the two bones actually possesses the "saddle" configuration? Close inspection will reveal that both articulating surfaces are of this form.

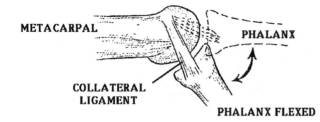

Figure 9:1 Collateral ligament action at the metacarpophalangeal joints of the finger.

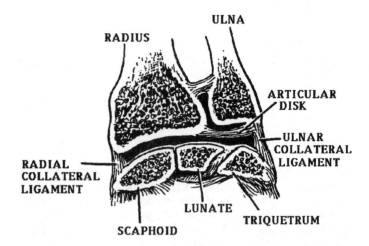

Figure 9:2 The radiocarpal and distal radioulnar joints.

Extension and flexion carry the thumb in a plane which is parallel with the palm; abduction and adduction move the thumb at right angles to the plane of the palm. "Opposition" enables one to touch the tip of the thumb to the tip of each of the fingers and involves a combination of movments including abduction, rotation, flexion, adduction and extension.

Expose the fibrous capsule which joins the trapezium and the metacarpal bone of the thumb, by excising adjacent tendons and tissues. Widely incise the articular capsule so that the articular bony surfaces can be inspected. Note the complexity of form of the articular faces of the two bones.

Anatomy of the Joints at the Wrist

Two primary joints - with a number of subparts - are involved in the architecture of the wrist. The more proximal joint is called the **radiocarpal joint**; more distal is the **midcarpal joint**. In addition to these, there are a number of individual intercarpal joints (which we will ignore, for the most part).

The Radiocarpal, or Wrist Joint. The radiocarpal joint is **elipsoidal** in form, and involves the articulation of the distal end of the radius and an articular disk, proximally, with the scaphoid, lunate and triquetral bones, distally. The distal radius articulates directly with the scaphoid and lunate bones; the articular disk - which joins the styloid process of the ulna and the medial edge of the distal radius together - articulates with the triquetrum. The structure of this joint is such that it allows flexion, extension, adduction, abduction and circumduction.

The capsule of the radiocarpal joint encloses the distal ends of the radius and ulna and extends to the scaphoid (navicular), lunate and triquetral bones (Fig. 9:2). **Note: The ulna does not articulate directly with any of the carpal bones of the wrist.** The capsule is reinforced by a number of fairly distinct ligaments - most of which can be seen and identified far more easily with an arthroscope than in the gross anatomy laboratory. Consequently, one will give these very little attention in the dissection; that is, unless you'd like to do a little additional work, independently.

Remember that pronation and supination are functions of the proximal and distal radio-ulnar joints. The radiocarpal joint, then, does not have an active role in these functions.

The Mid-Carpal Joint. The mid-carpal joint involves the articulation between the proximal row of carpal bones and the distal row of carpal bones. The proximal row includes the scaphoid, lunate and triquetral bones, with the pisiform situtated somewhat like a bystander to the action. The distal row is composed of the trapezium, trapezoid, capitate and hamate bones. This joint is somewhat mixed in type, including some features of an elipsoidal joint and of a plane joint. Important ligaments join the bones of the joint together and facilitate the smoothness of its normal movements.

*Divide the tendons which cross the dorsal surface of the wrist and then, using your scalpel and scissors (carefully) remove the part of the joint capsule which covers the bones articulating at the wrist. This will allow you to inspect the interior of the **radiocarpal (wrist) joint**, the **mid-carpal joint** and the **distal radio-ulnar joint**.*

*Identify the **articular disk** of the radiocarpal joint. Note that the disk separates the head of the ulna from direct articulation with the carpus. Observe that the articular disk binds the styloid* *process of the ulna with the medial edge of the distal end of the radius.*

In addition to its articulation with the ulna, the concave distal end of the radius is apposed to the convex surfaces of the **scaphoid** and **lunate bones.**

*At the lateral and medial aspects of the radio-carpal joint identify the **radial collateral ligament** and the **ulnar collateral ligament.** Anterior and posterior radiocarpal ligaments and intercarpal ligaments are also of significance in strengthening the wrist joint, but need not be dissected.*

Fracture of the scaphoid (navicular bone) is the most common injury to the carpal bones in falls upon the hand, producing swelling and pain in the area of the "anatomical snuff-box." Fracture of the distal metaphysis of the radius (**Colles' fracture**) is the most common fracture in adults over fifty years of age. Falling upon the open hand with the forearm pronated is the usual cause of such a fracture. The broken end of the radius is displaced posteriorly, producing a noticeable deviation just proximal to the wrist, resulting in the so-called "dinner-fork" deformity of the forearm and hand.

The Radio-Ulnar Joints

A Note: It can be a little difficult, initially, to see that the joints between the radius and ulna are three in number; that the most distal contributes to the appearance and function of the region of the wrist; that the intermediate joint is a little different in structure than most joints you will be asked to learn about, and that the proximal radio-ulnar joint is an important part of that region which we refer to, somewhat inaccurately, as the elbow joint.

The Distal Radio-ulnar Joint. The distal radio-ulnar joint is of the **trochoid** or pivot-type, the head of the ulna articulating with the **ulnar notch** of the distal end of the radius. The rotation of the distal end of the radius about the head of the ulna results in pronation and supination of the forearm. The two bones are held together distally by a number of ligamentous structures, the most important of which is the   the fibrocartilaginous **articular disk** which joins the two bones together and which serves to separate the distal end of the ulna from direct contact with the carpal bones.   Distally, the fibrocartilaginous disk is in contact with the **triquetral** bone and the medial part of the **lunate bone.**

The Middle Radio-Ulnar Joint. The middle radio-ulnar union is a **syndesmosis** formed principally by the interosseous membrane, which joins the shafts of the radius and ulna together. The orientation of the fibers of the interosseous membrane is obliquely downward and medial from the radius to the ulna, for the most part, although

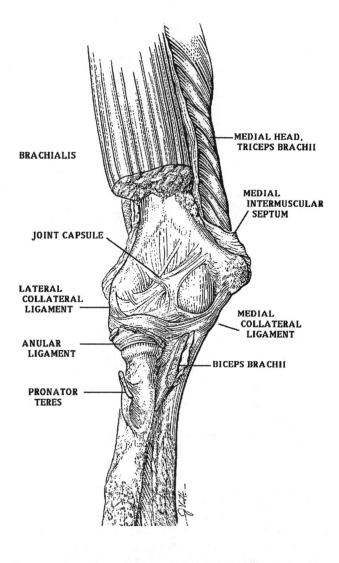

Figure 9:3 Anterior view of the region of the elbow joint.

some of the more dorsal fibers are oriented in the opposite plane.

The direction of the fibers of the membrane is of significance in transferral of forces between the radius, ulna and humerus. Can you see how? The ligamentous fibers pass mostly obliquely, medially, and distalward from the radius to the ulna. Forces applied to the hand are transferred upward through the wrist and then to the radius - carried then by the ulna. Thereafter, the humerus receives the impact through the humeral trochlea and the proximal part of the ulna.

*The internal features of the distal radio-ulnar joint are seen in the exposure of structures at the wrist. Preserving the nerves and arteries, as much as possible, strip away the musculature from the dorsum and ventral surface of the forearm and expose the **interosseous membrane** of the middle radio-ulnar union.*

148

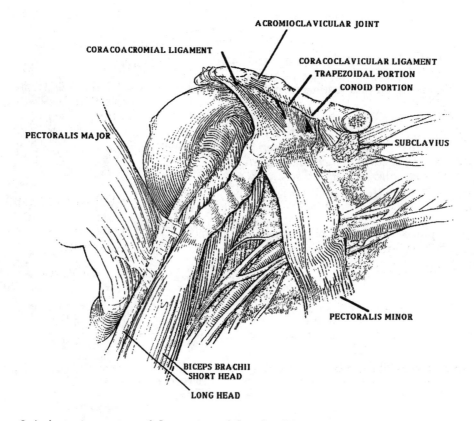

Figure 9:4 Anterior aspect of the region of the shoulder joint.

*Again identify the **common interosseous artery** and its **posterior interosseous branch**. Note the course of the **deep branch of the radial nerve** as it passes into, and through, the supinator muscle. Divide the biceps, brachialis and triceps at their insertions and reflect them away from the elbow. Also reflext the anconeus toward its ulnar insertion. Pronate and supinate the forearm to demonstrate the functions of the **proximal** and **distal radio-ulnar joints**.*

The Proximal Radio-Ulnar Joint. The proximal radio-ulnar joint is formed by the articulation between the head of the radius and the radial notch of the proximal end of the ulna. The proximal radio-ulnar joint is of the **trochoid** (pivot) type, making it possible to pronate and supinate the forearm. In addition to other capsular fibers, the joint depends upon the strength of the anular ligament which binds the two bones together. This ligament will be exposed as the elbow region is dissected.

Anatomy of the Joints at the Elbow

At the elbow, a common synovial membrane encloses the articulations of:
(1) the trochlea and capitulum of the humerus and their junctions with the semilunar notch of the ulna and head of the radius, respectively;

(2) the head of the radius and its junction with the radial notch of the ulna.

The articulation of the **semilunar notch** of the ulna with the **trochlea** of the humerus forms a hinge (**ginglymus**) joint. Note, however, that when you extend your forearm, the hand tends to move away from the midline of the extremity - due to the oblique contour of the trochlea - thus, the hinge does not function in a strictly antero-posterior plane.

The forearm is not in a straight line with the long axis of the humerus. The angle at which it meets the brachium at the elbow is called **the carrying angle**. This angle of deviation is greater in females than in males. Remember, in this context, that the ulnar nerve can be put under tension as it passes posteriorly around the medial epicondyle. The likelihood of this is greater as the carrying angle increases. The greater deviation of the carrying angle in women probably has an affect upon the frequency with which women have problems associated with ulnar nerve trauma.

*Before dissecting the region of the elbow, remove the muscles (**but not the nerves or vessels**) from around the elbow. After cutting and reflecting the tendon of the triceps, identify the posterior aspect of the articular capsule of the elbow joint. Remove a portion of the capsule to expose the **olecranon fossa** of the humerus, into which the tip of the **olecranon***

149

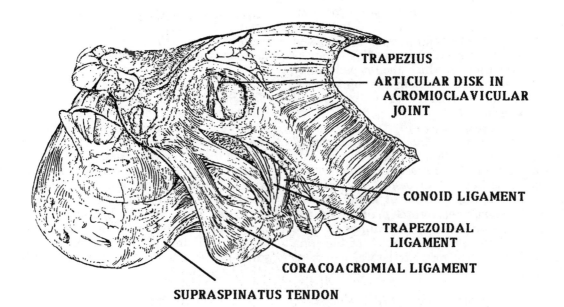

Figure 9:5 Superior view of the region of the right shoulder joint. The rounded head of the humerus is to the viewer's left.

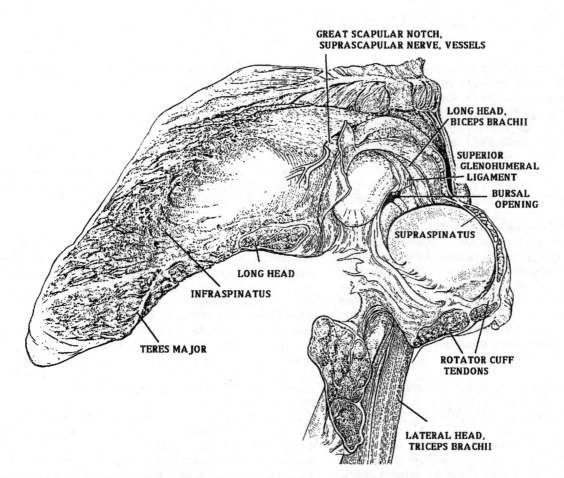

Figure 9:6 Posterior view of the right shoulder joint, opened from behind and with most muscles cut away.

150

process of the ulna glides in extension of the forearm. *Look for the* **fat pad** *in the joint.* It has a characteristic appearance on x-rays which can provide significant information regarding injuries there - such as fractures, in which the fat pad can be obviously displaced by blood within the joint cavity. The articular capsule is attached to the margins of the olecranon fossa.

Palpate the head of the radius and the coronoid process of the ulna and then incise the articular capsule just proximal to those processes. Enlarge the capsular incision sufficiently to inspect the internal bony features, identifying the **radial head, radial fossa of the humerus, coronoid process of the ulna** *and the* **coronoid fossa of the humerus.** The close adaptation of the semilunar notch of the ulna with the humeral trochlea restricts lateral movment of the elbow joint.

With a saw, transect the neck of the radius (between the head of the radius and the **bicipital tuberosity**). The strong, **anular ligament** normally confines the head of the radius in the radial notch of the ulna (Fig. 9:3). *Remove the head of the radius to inspect the attachments of the anular ligament.* **Alternatively,** *incise the anular ligament longitudinally to expose the internal features of the joint.*

Remember: The **proximal radial-ulnar articulation**, like its distal counterpart, is a pivot (**trochoid**) type joint.

By shaving away the tendinous origins of the flexor and extensor muscles, and the origin of the supinator attempt to identify the thickened lateral and medial portions of the articular capsule of the elbow joint - the **radial collateral** *and* **ulnar collateral ligaments.**

Articulations of Pectoral Girdle and Shoulder

The Acromioclavicular Joint. The **acromioclavicular joint** is formed between the lateral end of the clavicle and the acromion process of the scapula; it is important in circular movements of the scapula on the ribs. The capsule of this joint and the ligaments which suspend the scapula from the clavicle may be torn in the common "shoulder separation," or completely divided in a complete dislocation of the joint, from trauma to the top of the shoulder.

Demonstrate the features of the **acromioclavicular joint.** *Move the distal portion of the previously transected clavicle to show the position of junction of the clavicle with the acromion process. Note the fibers that bind the two bones together at this joint. Use your scalpel to shave away the dorsal part of the joint capsule. Is an articular disk present? It is in about 50% of individuals - at least partially (Fig. 9:4).*

Identify the **trapezoid** *and* **conoid** *portions of the* **coracoclavicular ligament** (Figs. 9:4, 5). These can be torn through in shoulder separations, necessitating surgical repair.

The Sternoclavicular Joint. The bony **pectoral girdle** consists of the clavicle and scapula. Numerous muscles are involved in the attachment of the pectoral girdle to the trunk; however, there is only one bony articulation, the **sternoclavicular joint**, formed by the articulation between the medial end of the clavicle and the manubrium of the sternum. The joint contains a very important **articular disk** which subdivides the joint, allowing for greater complexity of movments possible there. Like the MP joint of the thumb, this is also a **saddle joint** or, as some authorities refer to it, a **double gliding joint.**

The articular disk is attached about its circumference to the clavicle and the manubrium of the sternum by **anterior** and **posterior sternoclavicular ligaments** and by **interclavicular ligaments**, which are thickenings of the capsule. The disk is attached below to the cartilage of the first rib.

The articulation of the clavicle is further strengthened by the presence of the **costoclavicular ligament**. This short, rhomboid-shaped, stout ligament is situated just lateral to the capsule of the sternoclavicular joint and tethers the costal cartilage of the first rib to the inferior aspect of the medial end of the clavicle. This ligament limits elevation of the shoulder.

Make a shallow saw cut parallel with the clavicle through the sternoclavicular joint. **Alternatively,** *cut away the anterior part of the capsule to inspect the interior of the joint. Identify the* **articular disk.** *Note that the articular disk divides the joint into two separate cavities.*

Dissect away the origin of the **subclavius muscle** *and, deep to it, identify the* **costoclavicular ligament**.

The Glenohumeral Joint. The principal articulation of the upper limb is that between the glenoid fossa of the scapula and the head of the humerus. This is an **enarthrodial** (ball and socket) joint.

The **glenohumeral ligaments**, thickenings of the anterior part of the articular capsule of the joint, are of relatively little use in strengthening the shoulder joint or in preventing dislocation. The **superior glenohumeral ligament** is the most readily and consistently seen member of this group of ligaments (**superior, intermediate, inferior**). These ligaments are of more importance (at present in the clinical environment) by their usefulness in providing material for sutures to bite into to strengthen the capsule of the joint, in cases of chronic anterior dislocation of the shoulder.

Because the articular cavity of the shoulder is so shallow, it is frequently subject to ligamentous strains or tears, **subluxation** (partial separation of the humeral head from the glenoid fossa), or **dislocation** (luxation, complete separation of the two bony surfaces). The most significant factor in the maintenance of the stability of the shoulder joint is the muscular rotator cuff.

*Cut the pectoralis minor, the short head of the biceps and the coracobrachialis at their attachments to the coracoid process. This will facilitate the exposure of the anterior aspect of the **shoulder joint**. Identify the **subscapularis muscle** as it passes to insertion upon the lesser tuberosity of the head of the humerus. Transect the subscapularis about an inch from its insertion and then reflect the subscapularis posteriorly. Identify the **subscapularis bursa**, deep to the muscle.* This bursa frequently communicates with the capsule of the shoulder joint (Fig. 9:6). Some fibers of the subscapularis usually insert upon the capsule.

*Identify the **tendon of the long head of the biceps** in the **bicipital** (intertubercular) **groove** of the humerus.* This tendon is rather unique in that it passes through a joint. From its origin above the **glenoid fossa** of the scapula, the tendon passes through the shoulder joint (ensheathed in synovial membrane) and over the head of the humerus, thus tending to fix and steady the head of the humerus in the joint.

The subscapularis forms the medial portion of the **muscular rotator cuff** of the shoulder joint. The **supraspinatus, infraspinatus** and **teres minor** (the SIT group) form the lateral aspect of the rotator cuff. *Divide and reflect each of these muscles toward its insertion upon the greater tuberosity. Turn the body so that the posterior aspect of the shoulder can be seen. The posterior aspect of the capsule of the shoulder joint can now be exposed.*

*Incise and remove the posterior portion of the **articular capsule** of the shoulder joint. Rotate the head of the humerus medially out of the **glenoid cavity**. Identify the fibrocartilaginous **glenoid labrum** (which deepens the otherwise shallow articular cavity), the **glenoid cavity**, the tendon of the **long head of the biceps**, the **opening into the subscapularis bursa** and the **glenohumeral ligaments**.*

*Identify the **coracoacromial ligament**. Note the sharp lateral edge of this ligament. The supraspinatus tendon can be subject to severe damage by its contact with the ligament - particularly in strenuous activities - and be thus weakened or torn. Identify the **coracohumeral ligament**, if possible. This ligament leaves the coracoid process at a deeper plane than the coracoacromial ligament and passes into the capsule of the joint just anterior to the passage of the tendon of the supraspinatus muscle.*

QUESTIONS FOR REVIEW AND STUDY

1. What are the characteristics of a diarthrodial joint?

Bones covered with hyaline cartilage; lined with synovial membrane; possesses fibrous capsule continuous with periosteum; freely movable

2. What is the most freely movable diarthrosis?

The shoulder joint

3. What is the "weak area" of the articular capsule of the shoulder?

The inferior aspect, which has no musculotendinous reinforcement

4. What are the most important supportive features of the shoulder joint?

The muscles and tendons which invest its anterior, superior and posterior aspects

5. What muscles contribute to the "rotator cuff"?

Supraspinatus, infraspinatus, teres minor (all laterally); subscapularis (medially)

6. What ligament acts as an osseofibrous arch over the shoulder joint? What bursa is related to it? What tendon is associated which this bursa?

The coracoacromial ligament.
Between this arch and the shoulder fibrous capsule is the subacromial bursa. Supraspinatus tendon.

7. What is the most frequent type of shoulder dislocation? What is the second-most frequent? What are two other types of dislocations?

Subcoracoid-head of humerus lies beneath the coracoid process and the muscles which attach to the coracoid;
Subglenoid is second in frequency (both total 98% of occurrences).
Subclavicular and subspinous

8. What is the relationship of the long biceps tendon to the shoulder joint?

Passes through it, although covered with synovium and therefore extrasynovial in position; the only such tendon-joint relationship in the body.

9. What three joints contribute to the formation of the elbow joint?

Humero-ulnar; humero-radial; proximal radio-ulnar

10. What ligaments are present on either side of each interphalangeal joint? With what general type of joints are such ligaments associated?

Medial and lateral collateral ligaments. Collateral ligaments are found on either side of hinge-type joints (ginglymus joints).

11. Define and give examples of each of the following joint types (diarthroses already noted above):

a. Juncturae fibrosae (synarthrosis)

a. Immovable joints, in which the bones are joined by fibrous tissue or cartilage such as: (1) sutura, found in the skull; (2) gomphosis - articulations in socket, as for teeth; (3) syndesmosis, as in tibiofibular articulation, where bones are joined by interosseous ligaments; as also in the intercarpal joints of the wrist.

b. Synchondrosis

b. Bony surfaces joined by cartilage, as in epiphyseal junctions with long bones.

c. Symphysis

c. Bony surfaces joined by flattened plates of fibro-cartilage; as in intervertebral disks, pubic symphysis

d. Ginglymus

d. Hinge joint, interphalangeal joint, humero-ulnar joint

e. Trochoid

e. Pivot-joint; movement limited to rotation, as in the proximal radio-ulnar joint, where the head of the radius rotates within the fibrous anular ligament, and as in the articulation of the odontoid process of the axis with the atlas

f. Elipsoidal

f. An ovoid articular surface received into an elliptical cavity, like the radio-carpal articulation; permits all movements except axial rotation

g. Saddle joint

g. Reciprocal concave-convex bony surfaces movements as in condyloid joint; example is carpo-metacarpal joint of the thumb

h. Enarthrosis

h. Ball and socket; hip and shoulder joints

i. Arthrodia

i. Gliding joints; only movement permitted is gliding, as in joints between vertebral articular processes

12. With what bone does the humeral-

a. trochlea articulate?
b. capitulum articulate?

a. Ulna (trochlear or semilunar notch)
b. Radius (fovea of head)

13. With what bones does the radius articulate at the wrist?

With the ulna (the head of the ulna joins the ulnar notch of the radius); with the scaphoid and lunate bones

14. Does the ulna articulate directly with carpal bones?

No. It is separated from the carpus by the articular disk.

15. Name the bones in the proximal row of the carpus.

Scaphoid, lunate, triquetrum, pisiform

16. Name the bones in the distal row of the carpus.

Trapezoid, trapezium, capitate, hamate

17. What is the most commonly dislocated bone of the wrist (of the carpal bones). In what direction is this bone usually displaced? What is the clinical importance of this dislocation.

The lunate bone. Displacement is always anteriorly. Dislocation of the lunate bone can precipitate the signs associated typically with carpal tunnel syndrome.

154

LABORATORY IDENTIFICATION
CHECK-LIST

Articulations of The Upper Member

metacarpophalangeal (MP) joint

fibrous articular capsule

collateral ligaments of MP joint

proximal interphalangeal joint (PIP)
distal interphalangeal joint (DIP)

fibrous capsule of carpal-metacarpal joint of thumb
trapezium

radiocarpal joint

distal radio-ulnar joint
head of ulna
ulnar notch of radius

articular disk of radio-carpal joint
triquetrum
lunate bone

scaphoid bone

radial collateral ligament of radiocarpal joint
ulnar collateral ligament of radiocarpal joint

interosseous membrane
common interosseous artery
posterior interosseous artery
deep branch of radial nerve

proximal radio-ulnar joint

articular capsule of elbow joint

olecranon fossa
olecranon process

head of radius
radial fossa of humerus
coronoid process of ulna
coronoid fossa of humerus
neck of radius

bicipital tuberosity
anular ligament of head of radius
radial notch of ulna
radial collateral ligament of elbow
ulnar collateral ligament of elbow
acromioclavicular joint
articular disk of acromioclavicular joint
coracoclavicular ligament-trapezoid portion
coracoclavicular ligament-conoid portion

sternoclavicular joint
articular disk of sternoclavicular joint
anterior and posterior sternoclavicular ligaments
interclavicular ligaments
costoclavicular ligament

subscapularis muscle at insertion
subscapularis bursa
bicipital groove of humerus
tendon of long head of biceps
articular capsule of shoulder joint
glenohumeral ligaments

DEFINITIONS

Condyloid [Gr. *condyle*, knuckle + *eidos,* form]
   Resembling a condyle or knuckle.

Conoid - Resembling or shaped like a cone.

Diarthrosis [Gr. *dia*, through + *arthron*, joint]

Glenoid [Gr. *glene,* socket + *eidos* form]
   Resembling a pit or socket.

Olecranon[Gr. *olenee*, elbow + *kranion*, head]
   The head or tip of the elbow.

Synarthrosis [Gr. *sun*, with + *arthron*, joint]
   A fixed union of two bones.

Symphysis [Gr. *sun*, together + *physis*, a growing together]
   A union of two bones by fibrocartilage.

Trapezoid [Gr. *trapezoeides,* table shaped]
   Having the shape of a four-sided plane, with two sides parallel and two diverging.

Trochlea (pl. trochleae) [Gr. *trochilia,* pulley]
   A pulley-shaped part or structure.

Trochoid [Gr. *trochos*, wheel + *eidos*, resembling]
   A wheel-like articulation. A pivotal joint.

PART IV

THE LOWER LIMB

CHAPTER 10
THE THIGH
(ANTERIOR AND MEDIAL COMPARTMENTS)

Introduction

Study the articulated skeleton and other available osteological material to become acquainted with the bones that compose the skeleton of the lower extremity. For the first dissection give particular attention to the hip bone and the femur (Fig. 10:2, 3).

Upon yourself, and then upon the cadaver, palpate the following structures:

Anterior superior and posterior superior iliac spines
Pubic tubercles and pubic symphysis
Greater trochanter of the femur
Medial and lateral femoral condyles
Patella
Tibial tuberosity
Head and neck of the fibula
Medial and lateral malleoli of the ankle

Superficial Dissection

*Palpate the **medial malleolus**, then make a transverse skin incision just proximal to the malleolus and identify the **great saphenous vein.** Divide the skin and superficial fascia over the great saphenous vein from the ankle cephalically to the knee. Secure and clean the **saphenous nerve.***

The **saphenous nerve** first makes its appearance at the posteromedial aspect of the knee and accompanies the great saphenous vein to the medial side of the foot. Proximal to the knee the nerve is hidden by the sartorius muscle of the thigh. The saphenous nerve is the longest sensory branch of the femoral nerve and carries sensory fibers from the fourth lumbar nerve to the medial surface of the leg and foot (the **L4 dermatome** of the lower limb).

The great saphenous vein is frequently "harvested" (excised) for use in coronary bypass procedures (and for other surgical purposes). Patients often complain after the heart surgery that the pain which they feel on the medial side of the leg is greater than that experienced from the incision made in the chest. The anesthesia, pain or burning sensations present along the leg can be lessened, according to some surgeons if the vein is stripped downward from the knee toward the ankle - rather than the reverse direction - because of the anatomic relationship of the vein to the saphenous nerve.

Near the knee, the saphenous nerve lies deep to the vein, separated from it by a variable quantity of

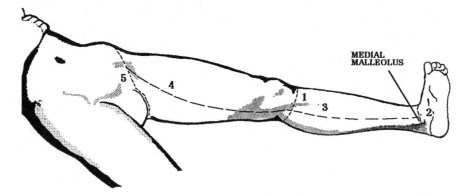

Figure 10:1 Initial incisions for exposure of great saphenous vein, saphenous nerve and reflection of the skin. 1, Transverse incision below knee. 2, Transverse incision at ankle. 3, Incision over great saphenous vein in leg; 4, in thigh. 5, Incision parallel with inguinal ligament, medially around genitalia.

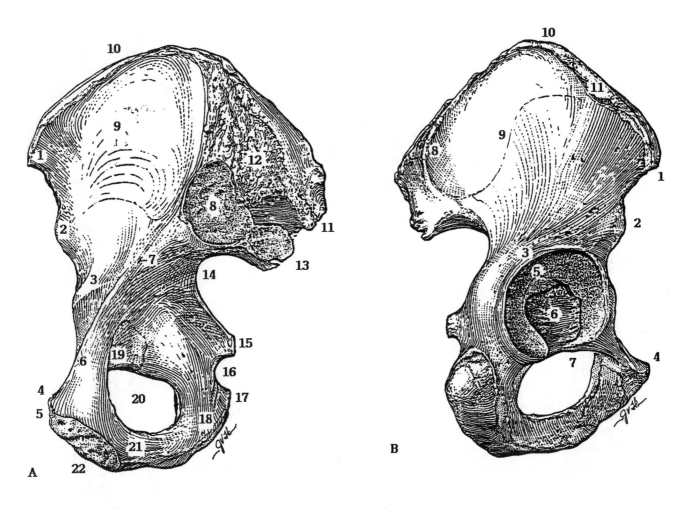

Figure 10:2 The os coxae (innominate) bone - viewed from its medial and lateral aspects.

A. Medial view

1. Anterior superior iliac spine
2. Anterior inferior iliac spine
3. Iliopectineal eminence
4. Pubic tubercle
5. Pubic crest
6. Pectineal line
7. Arcuate line
8. Auricular surface
9. Iliac fossa
10. Iliac crest
11. Posterior superior iliac spine
12. Roughened area for sacroiliac ligament
13. Posterior inferior iliac spine
14. Greater sciatic notch
15. Spine of the ischium
16. Lesser sciatic notch
17. Ischial tuberosity
18. Ramus of ischium
19. Groove for obturator vessels
20. Obturator foramen
21. Inferior ramus of pubis
22. Symphyseal surface

B. Lateral view

1. Anterior superior iliac spine
2. Anterior inferior iliac spine
3. Acetabular labrum
4. Pubic tubercle
5. Lunate surface
6. Acetabular fossa (non-articular area)
7. Acetabular notch
8. Posterior gluteal line
9. Anterior gluteal line
10. Iliac crest
11. Tubercle of the crest of the ilium

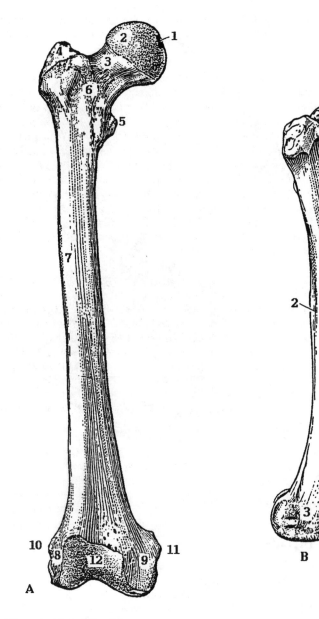
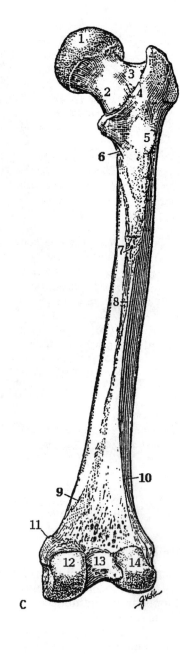

Figure 10:3 The Femur.

A. Ventral surface

1. Fovea capitis
2. Head
3. Neck
4. Greater trochanter
5. Lesser trochanter
6. Intertrochanteric line
7. Shaft
8. Lateral condyle
9. Medial condyle
10. Lateral epicondyle
11. Medial epicondyle
12. Patellar surface

B. Lateral view

1. Head
2. Linea aspera
3. Lateral condyle

C. Dorsal surface

1. Head
2. Neck
3. Trochanteric fossa
4. Intertrochanteric crest
5. Gluteal tuberosity
6. Pectineal line
7. Nutrient foramen of shaft
8. Linea aspera
9. Medial supracondylar line
10. Lateral supracondylar line
11. Adductor tubercle
12. Medial condyle
13. Intercondylar fossa
14. Lateral condyle

161

fat and connective tissue. More distally, the two structures come into closer relationship, with the nerve often giving off branches which pass close to, or over, tributaries to the vein. If the vein is removed from the ankle to the knee, there is a greater liklihood of avulsing (tearing) larger branches of the nerve, or even the saphenous nerve itself - resulting in the clinical signs described above.

The **great saphenous vein** arises from the medial aspect of the dorsal venous arch of the foot and terminates in the femoral vein. Appearances not withstanding, the great saphenous vein is comparable embryologically to the cephalic vein of the upper limb. If you imagine the lower limb rotated laterally so that the knee and the elbow point in the same direction you will begin to note some interesting similarities in the morphology of the two extremities. This orientation of the limbs is similar to that seen in the fetal condition.

Make a circumferential incision through the skin encompassing the leg just distal to the patella (to limit the initial skin reflection to the thigh and gluteal region). Look for the **infrapatellar branch** *of the* saphenous nerve in the subcutaneous tissues over the patellar ligament and patella.

Now divide the skin over the great saphenous vein up the medial aspect of the thigh to the **saphenous hiatus** *(Fig. 10:1).* The saphenous hiatus is an opening in the deep fascia through which the saphenous vein passes to drain into the femoral vein. *Do not disturb the delicate* **cribriform fascia** *which fills the saphenous hiatus; it will be removed somewhat later in the dissection.*

Note the numerous lymph nodes in the region just inferior to the inguinal ligament. These nodes are divided by their location relative to the deep fascia into **superficial** *and* **deep inguinal lymph nodes.**

The inguinal lymph nodes receive lymph from the entire lower limb, the gluteal region (buttocks), the perineum, the external genitalia (excluding the testes) and the lower anterior abdominal wall below the level of the umbilicus. In the female, some lymphatic drainage from the upper part of the uterus can pass along the lymphatic vessels of the round ligament, draining then into the inguinal nodes - a fact which can be of some diagnostic importance, when the uterus is diseased.

Superficial *and* **deep perforating tributaries** *to* the **great saphenous vein** *should be observed, for they are important, but do not preserve them.*

Abduct the thighs. Place an incision through the skin medially where the thigh joins the body, carrying this incision posteriorly around the genitalia. Leave the skin upon the external genitalia and in the area about the anus at this time. If the abdominal skin is still intact, it will be necessary to divide the skin over

the inguinal ligament upwards to the anterior superior iliac spine, taking great care not to cut the superficial vessels in the region.

Several small arteries arise typically from the proximal segment of the femoral artery as it enters the thigh. These vessels include the **superficial circumflex iliac, superficial epigastric and superficial external pudendal** artery. The superficial circumflex iliac passes laterally, just inferior to the inguinal ligament, to the region distal to the anterior superior iliac spine. The superficial epigastric artery passes vertically craniad, crossing to the anterior abdominal wall, near the mid-point of the inguinal ligament. The superficial external pudendal artery courses medially, into the superficial tissues of the genitalia.

Reflect the skin and **superficial fascia** *medially and laterally from the thigh as far as you can without turning the body over. Identify the* **superficial circumflex iliac, superficial epigastric and superficial external pudendal vessels**. *[In some individuals, one or more of these vessels may be so tiny - or even absent - so, do not spend a lot of time searching for them.* Note, and attempt to save, the cutaneous nerves of the thigh. Leave the deep fascia, the **fascia lata**, intact, to avoid damage to deeper structures.*

Observe the thickened lateral part of the fascia lata referred to as the **iliotibial tract**. The iliotibial tract is composed of tendinous fibers of the tensor fasciae latae muscle and the gluteus maximus muscle which are incorporated within the fascia lata - thickening it, and strengthening it. The iliotibial tract extends to

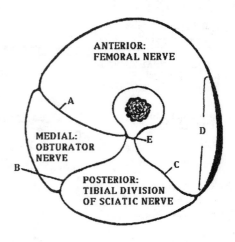

Figure 10:4 Schematic cross-section of the thigh

A = Medial intermuscular septum
B = Posterior intermuscular septum
C = Lateral intermuscular septum
D = Iliotibial tract
E = Linea aspera of femur

the lateral condyle of the tibia, inserting upon it, in part - contributing also to the dense lateral retinaculum at the knee. [The medial and lateral retinaculae of the knee consist of fascia lata, which are strengthened by additional fibrous tissue, including tendinous fibers from the more superficial muscles inserting in the area of the knee joint.]

Compartmentalization

The thigh can be conveniently divided into three compartments, each of which is associated with a principal nerve for motor supply of the muscles within (Fig. 10:4):
1.   Anterior chamber of the thigh (**extensor compartment**)
     Contents: quadriceps femoris muscle;
           sartorius muscle
     Nerve: femoral nerve
2.   Medial chamber of the thigh (**adductor compartment**)
     Contents: adductor longus, brevis and
           magnus;
           gracilis muscle;
           pectineus muscle
     Nerve: obturator nerve
3.   Posterior chamber of the thigh (**flexor compartment**)
     Contents: biceps femoris muscle;
           semitendinosus muscle;
           semimembranosus muscle
     Nerve: tibial division of sciatic nerve

Exceptions to these generalizations will be noted as you study further. For instance, the pectineus is supplied by the femoral nerve (usually); the adductor magnus is supplied both by the obturator nerve and the tibial division of the sciatic nerve; also, the short head of the biceps femoris is supplied by the peroneal division of the sciatic nerve.

Exposure of the Peritoneal Cavity.

Note to Students: The following dissection will be performed in order to help you visualize and understand the origin of many of the nerves and vessels which enter the thigh and the gluteal region from the abdominopelvic cavity.

Using the scalpel carefully, to avoid cutting the abdominal viscera,
(1) make a parasaggital incision through the body wall from approximately two-three inches above the umbilicus to the pubic bone. From the lower end of the vertical incision
(2) cut laterally along the pubic crest (on both sides of the body).
3) Incise the tissues over the course of the inguinal ligament to the anterior superior iliac spine.
(4) Make a transverse incision from the upper end of the vertical incision laterally to the midaxillary line.
(5)   Reflect the flaps of the anterior abdominal wall laterally. Push aside the abdominal viscera to observe   the   structures   which   arise   in   the

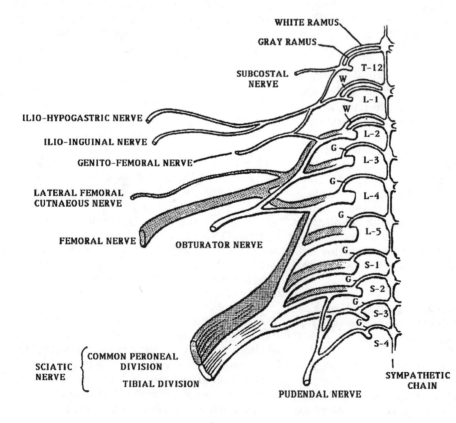

Figure 10:5 Constituents and branches of the lumbar and sacral plexuses. Nerves to extensor (posterior) muscles are shaded.

163

abdominopelvic cavity and pass into the thigh. It will be necessary to strip away the parietal peritoneum and fascia covering the nerves of the lumbosacral plexus, the iliac vessels and the posterior abdominal wall muscles.

Dissection of Abdominopelvic Structures

Muscles of the Posterior wall. *Identify and clean the muscles of the posterior abdominal wall which pass into the anterior thigh. Medially, the **psoas major** arises from the transverse processes and bodies of the lower thoracic and lumbar vertebrae. In about sixty percent of people, the tendon of a **psoas minor** muscle will be seen upon the psoas major.*

The iliacus muscle occupies the **iliac fossa**. The tendon of the iliacus joins that of the psoas major, passes beneath the inguinal ligament, and then inserts upon the proximal portion of the femur (on the lesser trochanter of the femur).

*Inferiorly, clean the fascia iliaca from the surface of the **iliacus muscle**, being carefull not to damage the nerves which pass inferiorly deep to, or within, this fascia.*

The Lumbar Plexus. *The ventral primary rami which enter into the formation of the lumbar nerve plexus will now be exposed (Fig. 10:5). First, palpate the twelfth rib and expose the **subcostal** (twelfth thoracic) **nerve** as it passes parallel with the inferior border of that rib.*

*Now, identify the **genitofemoral nerve** (L1, L2) as it passes superficially upon the psoas major muscle. Trace the nerve superiorly through the substance of the psoas to the origin of the nerve from the first and second **lumbar spinal nerves**.*

The **genitofemoral nerve** is sensory to the skin of the scrotum or labia majora, and also to a small region of skin inferior to the inguinal ligament, over the area of the femoral sheath. The genitofemoral nerve gives off skeletal motor nerve fibers to the cremaster muscle of the spermatic cord.

*On one side of the body carefully dissect the **psoas major muscle** in piecemeal fashion, preserving the lumbar nerves (which pass posterior to, or through, the psoas). Clean and identify the nerves which arise from the lumbar plexus:*
   *the **ilioinguinal nerve** (L1);*
   *the **genitofemoral nerve** (L1, 2);*
   *the **lateral femoral cutaneous nerve** (L2, 3);*
   *the **femoral nerve** (L2, 3, 4);*
   *the **obturator nerve** (L2, 3, 4);*
   *and the **lumbosacral trunk** (L4, 5).*

The ilioinguinal nerve is sensory to the skin of the upper, medial, thigh area and also to the scrotum and penis, or to labia majora.

The **obturator nerve** is composed of anterior divisions of the ventral primary rami from the second, third and fourth lumbar nerves; the **femoral nerve** is derived from the coalescence of the posterior divisions of these rami. Remember that anterior divisions of ventral primary rami supply muscles on the original (embryologic) ventral surface of the limb bud (flexors, adductors); the posterior divisions supply the dorsal (extensor) side of the limb.

*Identify the descending limb of the fourth lumbar nerve, the ventral ramus of the fifth lumbar nerve and their junction to form the **lumbosacral trunk**. The lumbosacral trunk and the ventral rami of the first four sacral nerves take part in the formation of the sacral plexus. Notice that the **sciatic nerve** arises from lumbar roots L4 and L5 and sacral roots S1, 2 and 3 (Fig. 10:5).*

*Trace the femoral nerve from its origin to the inguinal ligament. Also follow the **lateral femoral cutaneous nerve** to its passage beneath the inguinal ligament just medial to the anterior superior iliac spine.* The lateral femoral cutaneous nerve is implicated rather often in a clinical condition known as meralgia paresthetica, due to compression of the nerve as it passes deeply, beneath the inguinal ligament. You will read more about this shortly.

Iliac Vessels. At about the level of the fourth lumbar vertebra (i.e. slightly below the level of the umbilicus) the aorta divides into **right and left common iliac arteries**. These arteries pass on either side of the brim of the true pelvis, soon dividing into **external iliac** and **internal iliac** arteries. The **right** and **left common iliac veins** are formed by the confluence of the **internal** and **external iliac veins**. Subsequently, the right and left common iliac veins meet posterior to, and to the right side of the right common iliac artery, forming the beginning of the **inferior vena cava**. *Identify and clean the arteries and veins described.*

*Clean the **external iliac artery** and **vein** to their passage beneath the inguinal ligament. Identify the **deep circumflex iliac artery** and **vein**.* The deep circumflex iliac vessels may play a role in collateral circulation about the hip. Distal to the inguinal ligament the external iliac artery and vein are renamed the **femoral artery** and **vein**. *Just inferior to the ligament once more identify the **superficial circumflex iliac** and **superficial epigastric artery** and **vein**.*

Within the pelvis, the internal iliac artery divides into an **anterior division** and **a posterior division**. Three arterial branches commonly arise from the posterior division, the iliolumbar artery, one or two lateral sacral branches, and - the largest of its branches - the **superior gluteal artery**. The superior gluteal artery can usually be seen passing

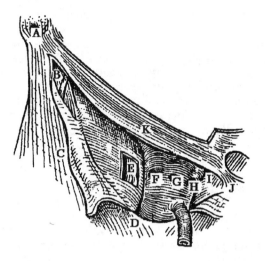

Figure 10:6 The femoral nerve, femoral sheath and associated structures.

A = Anterior superior iliac spine
B = Lateral femoral cutaneous nerve
C = Fascia reflected from inguinal ligament
D = Edge of saphenous hiatus
E = Femoral nerve, seen through window cut in fascia of iliopsoas muscle
F = Femoral artery
G = Femoral vein
H = Femoral canal
I = Transversalis fascia
J = Lacunar ligament - insertion of inguinal ligament (Position shown schematically only; it actually lies more deeply)
K = External oblique aponeurosis

deeply between the lumbosacral trunk and the first sacral nerve.

The anterior division of the internal iliac artery gives off a number of visceral branches (which need not be identified), before terminating by dividing into an internal pudendal branch and the large **inferior gluteal artery**. The inferior gluteal artery typically passes deeply between the first and second, or the second and third sacral nerves. As their names imply, the superior and inferior gluteal arteries provide the primary sources of arterial supply to the gluteal region. They will be seen again in the dissection of that area.

*Identify and clean the **iliolumbar artery**, the **lateral sacral artery** (ies) and the **superior gluteal artery**. Identify and clean the **obturator artery**, most commonly a branch of the anterior division of the internal iliac artery. [In more than 25% of individuals, however, the obturator artery arises from a branch of the <u>external iliac artery</u> just before it passes deep to the inguinal ligament.*

*By retracting the internal iliac artery and vein, attempt to visualize and expose the **inferior gluteal artery**.* This is (usually) one of the two major terminal branches of the anterior division. The other terminal branch, which you need not identify, is the internal pudendal artery. *Remove any venous vessels in the pelvis which obstruct your view.*

Sympathetic Supply of the Inferior Member. Each of the ventral rami which join the lumbar and sacral plexuses receives postganglionic sympathetic (gray communicating) rami from the abdominal or pelvic portions of the sympathetic chains (Fig. 10:5). The first two lumbar spinal nerves contribute preganglionic sympathetic (white communicating) rami to the sympathetic chains.

Vasospastic disorders of the lower limbs can at times be ameliorated by temporary pharmacological block at selected lumbar vertebral levels (sympathetic block). Surgical excision of lumbar sympathetic ganglia with their rami communicantes (sympathectomy) at lumbar levels two and three results in longer term relief. The first lumbar ganglion is frequently spared in lumbar sympathectomy of young adult males to avoid deletion of autonomic pathways essential for normal sexual activity.

Dissection of the Anterior Aspect of the Thigh

The Femoral Sheath, Femoral Hernia. *As you clean the external iliac vessels towards the inguinal ligament, note that they lie superficial to the fascia which covers the psoas and iliacus muscles, fascia which is named **fascia iliaca** in this position.* The fascia iliaca is, in reality, continuous with the **fascia transversalis** which covers the inner surface of the abdominal wall muscles, but the fascia is named according to the muscle with which it is associated. The two fasciae, then, are continuous (like a pleural "reflection") with one another at the inguinal ligament.

As the external iliac artery and vein pass beneath the inguinal ligament (becoming "femoral") they carry a prolongation of the fascial sheet provided by the fascia iliaca-transversalis. This fascial, tube-like investment of the vessels is named the **femoral sheath**. Leave the sheath intact for now.

The femoral sheath possesses three compartments with intervening fibrous septa - one for the femoral artery, one for the femoral vein, and a third compartment containing lymphatics, the **femoral canal** (Fig. 10:6).

*Medial to the femoral vein identify the **femoral ring**, the opening from the abdominal cavity into the femoral canal.* The ring is bounded medially by transversalis fascia and aponeurotic fibers of the transversus abdominis muscle passing to the pectineal (Cooper's) ligament, a stout ligamentous band on the pubic bone.

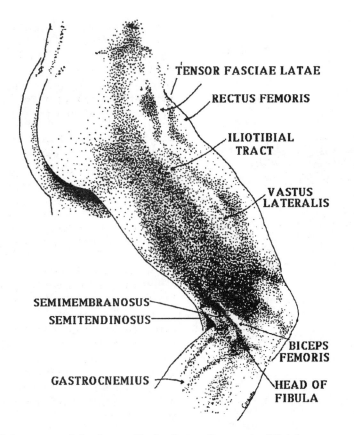

Figure 10:7 Superficial features of the lower limb - lateral aspect of thigh.

The femoral ring is bounded laterally by the fascia covering the femoral vein; anteriorly the ring is limited by the inguinal ligament; posteriorly the pubic bone limits the femoral ring. The femoral ring is usually occupied by a deep femoral lymph node (the "node of Cloquet"), together with numerous lymph vessels from the lower extremity.

The significance of the femoral ring lies in the etiology of **femoral hernias**. The herniating mass of extra-peritoneal fat, peritoneum and, variably, omentum and viscus pass through the femoral ring into the femoral canal. The hernia appears as a swelling lateral and inferior to the pubic tubercle (thus, differentiating it from an inguinal hernia), by passing through the **saphenous hiatus.** The saphenous hiatus, or fossa ovalis, is the opening in the fascia lata through which the great **saphenous vein** enters the femoral vein.

Removal of Fascia, Sensory Supply. *Distal to the inguinal ligament make a short longitudinal incision through the **fascia lata** (deep fascia of the thigh) over the femoral nerve. Protect the nerve by placing a probe deep to the inguinal ligament over the nerve before making the fascial incision. Similarly, expose the **lateral femoral cutaneous nerve**, which passes deep to the inguinal ligament, near the anterior superior iliac spine (Fig. 10:6).*

Meralgia Paresthetica. A rather common, although not usually grave disorder, occurs with compression of the lateral femoral cutaneous nerve where it passes deep to the inguinal ligament. Typically, the affected individual complains of burning, tingling or anesthesia on the proximal, lateral aspect of the thigh. The problem might first be noticed as a person puts a hand in the trouser pocket on the affected side and becomes aware of an uncomfortable sensation in the thigh where the fingertips touch it.

The causes of meralgia paresthetica are diverse. Sometimes it affects policemen who wear heavy pistol belts, workmen who wear heavy tool belts; persons in the latter stages of pregnancy, or who become obese or, conversely, have undergone rapid, severe weight loss. Anesthesia or pain of the thigh along the region of distribution of the lateral femoral cutaneous nerve can be noted by one who wears bluejeans which are too tight, or after having someone else sit on one's lap for a long period of time (!). Diabetic individuals may, apparently, be even more prone to such problems because of the sensitivity of the compressed nerves (or the blood supply of the nerves).

After locating the femoral and lateral femoral cutaneous nerves deep to the inguinal ligament, remove the fascia lata and muscular fascia from the muscles of the anterior and medial compartments of

166

the thigh. **Do not remove the iliotibial tract with the fascia lata.** The sensory supply of the anterior and lateral aspects of the thigh is provided by branches of the femoral nerve anteriorly and, laterally, by the lateral femoral cutaneous nerve.

The Sartorius Muscle. *Identify the sartorius muscle and clean it from its origin (at the anterior superior iliac spine) to the knee.* By virtue of its attachments the sartorius flexes the thigh and the leg and rotates the thigh laterally. *Transect the sartorius and reflect it, dividing its neural and vascular supply, if necessary.*

Femoral Triangle. The sartorius muscle forms the **lateral boundary** of an area called the **femoral triangle.** The **base** of the triangle is provided by the inguinal ligament, the **medial boundary** by the adductor longus muscle. The **apex** of the triangle is found at the intersection of the sartorius and adductor longus muscles. The triangle contains the femoral sheath, its contents, and the femoral nerve. The **floor** of the triangle is muscular and is formed by the iliopsoas and pectineus muscles.

Subsartorial Canal. *Within the femoral triangle reidentify the femoral sheath and the femoral nerve. [Note that the femoral nerve is **not within** the sheath].* At the **apex** of the femoral triangle the femoral artery and vein pass into the **subsartorial canal** (adductor canal, "Hunter's canal"). The femoral vessels remain in this canal until, near the knee, they pass through a hiatus in the tendon of the adductor magnus muscle to the posterior aspect of the knee. Subsequent to their passage through the adductor hiatus the vessels are renamed the **popliteal artery** and **vein.**

Dissection of Anterior Compartment. *Three small arteries arise from the initial segment of the femoral artery. These are the **superficial circumflex iliac, superficial epigastric** and **superficial external pudendal arteries.** Identify and clean these arteries.*

Incise the femoral sheath over the femoral artery and vein and open the femoral canal. Inspect the vessels, noting that within the femoral sheath the artery is situated lateral to the vein and courses beneath the midpoint of the inguinal ligament. The femoral nerve, in turn, lies lateral to the femoral artery and deep to the fascia iliaca.

*Dissect away the fascia that covers the femoral vessels, beginning at the inguinal ligament. Trace the vessels into the subsartorial canal and to the adductor hiatus. Near the proximal end of the canal identify the **nerve to the vastus medialis,** one of the important motor branches of the femoral nerve. Identify and preserve the **saphenous nerve** within the subsartorial canal. Trace the nerve to its origin from the femoral nerve and to its departure from the*

canal at the level of the knee. The saphenous nerve provides sensory supply to the knee, the medial aspect of the leg and the medial side of the foot - as noted earlier.

The Quadriceps Femoris. The quadriceps femoris muscle consists of four separate muscles which insert by the common quadriceps tendon upon the patella. The four heads of this muscle are named the **rectus femoris, vastus lateralis, vastus intermedius** and **vastus medialis.** All four of these muscles and the sartorius receive motor supply from the femoral nerve.

Note the origins of the four individual heads of the quadriceps femoris. The three "vasti" arise from the femur, whereas the rectus femoris (Fig. 10:7) originates partially from the anterior inferior iliac spine, partially from the brim of the acetabulum. Because of its attachments the rectus femoris flexes the thigh at the hip joint and, with the remainder of the quadriceps, also extends the knee.

The quadriceps tendon inserts upon the patella; the patella is anchored to the tuberosity of the tibia by the **ligamentum patella.** By its position and mobility the patella contributes to the mechanical advantage of the quadriceps tendon in extension of the knee. The patella is considered to be a **sesamoid bone** (a bone that develops in a tendon) because it is situated within the tendon of insertion of the quadriceps upon the tibia.

*Identify the nerve supply of the rectus femoris. Transect the rectus femoris distal to its innervation and reflect the muscle inferiorly. Deep to the divided rectus femoris identify the **vastus intermedius.***

Circumflex Arteries and Profunda Femoris. *Within the fascia that covers the proximal portion of the vastus intermedius identify and clean the **lateral femoral circumflex artery.** The **descending branch** of this artery leads directly into the **vastus lateralis** muscle and affords a plane of cleavage between the vastus intermedius and vastus lateralis.*

*Identify the branches of the **lateral femoral circumflex** artery upon the vastus intermedius. Trace any one of these proximally until the **lateral femoral circumflex** and its origin from the femoral artery or profunda femoris are clearly exposed.*

Attempt to identify the three branches of the lateral femoral circumflex: (1) The **descending branch** - passes deeply, between the vastus lateralis and vastus intermedius, and ultimately participates in the anastomoses about the knee; (2) the **transverse branch** - turns posteriorly below the greater trochanter of the femur and enters the vastus lateralis; (3) the **ascending branch** - courses more superiorly and anastomoses with several vessels

167

about the hip, including the deep circumflex iliac and superior gluteal arteries.

When the origin of the lateral femoral circumflex is seen it should be a relatively simple matter to identify the two other highly important branches of the femoral artery - the **profunda femoris** and **medial femoral circumflex** arteries - for they arise closely adjacent from the femoral artery. Indeed, all three arteries can arise from a common stem, separately, or in any combination with one another within two inches from the inguinal ligament. This can prove important in "cut-downs," or placement of ligatures, etc. of the femoral artery (or the femoral vein).

*Mobilize the **medial femoral circumflex artery** and clear away fascia to demonstrate the passage of the artery between the iliopsoas muscle and the **pectineus muscle**.*

*Clean the **profunda femoris** (deep femoral) artery from its origin to its disappearance distally, deep to the **adductor longus muscle**.* Several **perforating branches**, typically four, arise from the profunda femoris and pass medially about the femur to enter the posterior muscular compartment. The perforating arteries provide the principal sources of blood supply to the posterior chamber of the thigh. Their demonstration is optional in the dissection. The perforating tributaries to the **profunda femoris vein** constitute the major routes for venous drainage from the posterior chamber of the thigh to the femoral vein.

*At the **apex of the femoral triangle** confirm that a piercing wound may divide four vessels, from superficial to deep: the femoral artery, femoral vein, profunda femoris vein, profunda femoris artery.* This type of wound has been called the "butcher's thigh" injury, involving accidents with cleavers or other sharp instruments, resulting in rapid exsanguination and sometimes death.

The Cruciate Anastomosis. The so-called "cruciate" anastomosis classically involves the confluence of four arteries posterior to the upper part of the femur: (1) the transverse branch of the lateral femoral circumflex; (2) the medial femoral circumflex; (3) the descending branch of the inferior gluteal; (4) the ascending branch of the first perforating artery.

In actuality, the transverse branch of the lateral femoral circumflex may be very small or absent. Its ascending branch appears to participate more extensively in the anastomosis. Anastomoses about the hip also significantly involve such other vessels as the superior gluteal, iliolumbar, deep circumflex iliac, ascending branch of the lateral circumflex and the obturator artery. Many possible routes can therefore be available for collateral circulation from the iliac arteries to the extremity in occlusion of the femoral artery.

The Medial Compartment of the Thigh. *Deep, and lateral to the femoral artery identify the **iliopsoas muscle**.* The combined tendons of the two muscles insert upon the lesser trochanter; they therefore flex the thigh at the hip joint and rotate it, but they may also assist in flexing the trunk upon the thigh, as in "sit-ups".

The relationship of the femoral vessels and femoral nerve to the iliopsoas muscle is important in surgery upon the hip. The iliopsoas lies just between these structures and the anterior aspect of the capsule of the hip joint. The vessels and nerves are vulnerable to injury in operative procedures upon the hip (for instance, as when a pin driven into the neck of the femur is directed too far anteriorly).

*Just medial to the iliopsoas identify the **pectineus muscle**. [The medial femoral circumflex artery passes deeply in the interval between the two muscles].*

The pectineus arises from the superior pubic ramus and inserts upon the pectineal line of the femur, inferior to the lesser trochanter. The pectineus flexes, adducts and medially rotates the thigh at the hip joint. It is innervated usually by the femoral nerve, but occasionally receives supply from the **accessory obturator nerve**.

*Identify and clean the **gracilis muscle**. Note its innervation from the **anterior division of the obturator nerve**.* This muscle adducts the thigh. It inserts upon the tibia, however, and in paralysis of the "hamstrings" it may, with the assistance of the sartorius, assume the function of flexion of the knee.

*Clean the **adductor longus**. Transect the adductor longus at its origin from the front of the pubis, as close to the bone as possible. Reflect the muscle toward the femur.*

*Deep to the adductor longus, first identify the **anterior division of the obturator nerve**, then the **adductor brevis**.* The adductor longus and brevis are innervated by the anterior division of the obturator nerve.

*The adductor brevis should now be severed at its origin from the **inferior ramus** of the pubis and reflected to expose the **posterior division of the obturator nerve** and the great muscle it innervates, the **adductor magnus**.*

The adductor magnus is doubly innervated; that is, it is supplied both by the obturator nerve and by rami from the tibial division of the sciatic nerve. The adductor magnus inserts broadly upon the femur. Although it is principally a powerful adductor, different portions of the muscle can flex, extend, and medially or laterally rotate the thigh. Distal to its long insertion upon the linea aspera of the femur, the adductor magnus also inserts upon the adductor tubercle of the medial femoral condyle. The femoral artery and vein pass through an opening in the tendon of the adductor magnus between the linea aspera and the adductor tubercle, the **hiatus of the adductor magnus.** *Identify the **adductor hiatus.***

The obturator nerve gives off important articular branches to the hip and knee joints, in addition to its role in supplying the adductor musculature. Because of the articular branches, pain from pathologic processes may be "referred" from the hip to the region of the knee (and from the pelvis to the knee).

*Reflect the pectineus from the pubis and then identify the obturator artery and nerve at their appearance from the obturator foramen. Also identify the **obturator externus muscle.** Reflect the proximal part of the adductor magnus, if necessary, to expose the obturator externus adequately.* The tendon of this muscle passes posterior to the neck of the femur and inserts in the trochanteric fossa. It rotates the thigh laterally.

*Review the boundaries and contents of the subsartorial canal: (1) Its **roof**-sartorius; (2) **posterior wall** - adductor longus, adductor magnus; (3) **anterolateral wall** - vastus medialis; (4) it contains the femoral artery and vein, saphenous nerve, and the nerve to the vastus medialis.*

THE THIGH

MUSCLE	ORIGIN	INSERTION	ACTIONS	INNERVATION*
Iliopsoas	Iliac fossa; transverse processes and bodies of lumbar vertebrae	Lesser trochanter of femur	Flexes thigh at hip	Femoral nerve; direct branches from L1, L2
Sartorius	Anterior superior iliac spine	Pes anserinus - medial proximal tibia	Flexes thigh at hip; rotates thigh laterally; flexes knee	Femoral nerve (L2, L3)
Rectus Femoris	Anterior inferior iliac spine; superior lip, acetabulum	Patella; tibial tuberosity	Flexes thigh; extends knee	Femoral nerve (L2, L3)
Vastus Lateralis	Lateral aspect femur, linea aspera	Patella; tibial tuberosity	Extends knee	Femoral nerve (L2, L3)
Vastus Intermedius	Anterior aspect of femur	Patella; tibial tuberosity	Extends knee	Femoral nerve (L2, L3)
Vastus Medialis	Medial aspect of femur	Patella; tibial tuberosity	Extends knee - especially last 15 degrees	Femoral nerve (L2, L3)
Pectineus	Pubic pecten	Pectineal line of femur	Flexes and adducts thigh at hip	Femoral nerve (L2, L3)
Gracilis	Body of pubic bone	Pes anserinus - medial proximal tibia	Adducts thigh; flexes knee	Obturator nerve (anterior division, L2, L3)
Adductor Longus	Body of pubic bone	Linea aspera of femur	Adducts and flexes thigh at hip joint	Obturator nerve (Anterior division L2, L3)
Adductor Brevis	Inferior ramus of pubic bone	Linea aspera of femur	Adducts and flexes thigh at hip joint	Obturator nerve (anterior division, L2, L3)
Adductor Magnus	Inferior ramus of pubic bone; ischium, ischial tuberosity	Linea aspera; adductor tubercle	Adducts, extends, flexes, rotates thigh at hip joint	Obturator nerve (posterior division, L2, L3); tibial nerve (L5)

*In this column is listed the nerve innervating the given muscle, together with the principal spinal nerve roots involved in the <u>motor</u> supply of the muscle.

THE THIGH

MUSCLE	ORIGIN	INSERTION	ACTIONS	INNERVATION*
Biceps Femoris - long head	Ischial tuberosity	Head of fibula	Extends hip; flexes knee	Tibial nerve (L5)
Biceps Femoris - short head	Linea aspera of femur	Head of fibula	Flexes knee	Common peroneal nerve (S1)
Semimembranosus	Ischial tuberosity	Medial condyle of tibia, posteriorly	Extends hips; flexes knee	Tibial nerve (L5)
Semitendinosus	Ischial tuberosity	Pes anserinus, proximal medial tibia	Extends hip; flexes knee	Tibial nerve (L5)

*In this column is listed the nerve innervating the given muscle, together with the principal spinal nerve roots involved in the <u>motor</u> supply of the muscle.

QUESTIONS FOR REVIEW AND STUDY

1. Match the muscle with the nerve by which it is supplied motor fibers:

   1) Sartorius
   2) Rectus femoris
   3) Vastus intermedius
   4) Vastus lateralis
   5) Vastus medialis
   6) Pectineus
   7) Gracilis
   8) Adductor longus
   9) Adductor brevis
   10) Adductor magnus
   11) Obturator externus
   12) Semitendinosus
   13) Semimembranosus
   14) Long head, biceps femoris
   15) Short head, biceps femoris

   A. Tibial division, sciatic nerve
   B. Common peroneal division, sciatic nerve
   C. Obturator, anterior division
   D. Obturator, posterior division
   E. Femoral

   1 - 6. E (The pectineus may also be supplied by the accessory obturator nerve.)

   7 & 8. C
   9. C or D
   10. A, D
   11. D
   12 - 14. A
   15. B

2. What muscles seen in the thigh cross more than one joint, from origin to insertion?

   a. In the anterior compartment?

   b. In the medial compartment?

   c. In the posterior compartment?

   Of what importance is the above?

   a. Sartorius, rectus femoris

   b. Gracilis

   c. Semitendinosus, semimembranosus, long head of biceps femoris

   Such muscles exert their effects upon more than one joint.

3. The boundaries of the femoral triangle are:
   The base _____
   Lateral boundary _____
   Medial boundary _____

   Inguinal ligament
   Sartorius
   Adductor longus (lateral border of adductor longus)

4. Place the following in proper order from lateral to medial:
   a. Femoral canal
   b. Femoral nerve
   c. Femoral vein
   d. Femoral artery

   b, d, c, a

5. From what fascial layers is the femoral sheath derived?

   Fascia transversalis and fascia iliaca

172

6. What are the boundaries of the femoral ring?
   a. Medial

   b. Lateral
   c. Anterior
   d. Posterior

   a. Aponeurosis and fascia of the transversus abdominis muscle
   b. Fascia covering femoral vein
   c. Inguinal ligament
   d. Superior ramus of pubic bone

7. The subsartorial canal begins at __(a)__ and ends at __(b)__.

   a. Apex of femoral triangle
   b. Adductor hiatus

   c. Roof of the adductor canal:

   c. Sartorius

   d. Posterior wall:

   d. Adductor longus and magnus

   e. Anterolateral wall:

   e. Vastus medialis

   f. Contents of Hunter's canal:

   f. Femoral artery and vein, saphenous nerve, nerve to vastus medialis

8. The arterial supply of the posterior chamber of the thigh is provided by __(a)__, its venous drainage by __(b)__.

   a. Perforating branches of profunda femoris artery
   b. Perforating tributaries to profunda femoris vein

9. Diagram the "cruciate" anastomosis.

   1. Descending branch, inferior gluteal
   2. Medial femoral circumflex
   3. Ascending branch, lateral femoral circumflex
   4. Ascending branch, first perforating

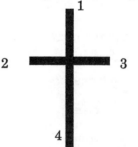

10. Trace several possible routes of collateral flow to the femoral artery in the event of occlusion of the external iliac at the inguinal ligament.

    Example 1: Internal iliac, inferior gluteal, medial femoral circumflex, femoral or profunda femoris

    Example 2: Internal iliac, inferior gluteal, first perforating, profunda, femoral

11. At what point does a femoral hernia leave the abdomen?

    Through the femoral ring, into the femoral canal. It emerges through the saphenous hiatus.

12. What structures must be incised to reach a herniating viscus at the saphenous hiatus?

    Skin, superficial fascia

13. What are the primary spinal nerve sources of motor supply to the quadriceps femoris and adductor muscles?

    L2 and L3

14. What spinal nerve carries the sensory fibers (monosynaptic) for the patellar reflex?

    L4

15. What nerve supplies the region of the L4 dermatome of the medial aspect of the leg and foot?

    Saphenous nerve

16. What spinal nerve levels predominate in the motor supply to the principal flexors of the hip joint?

    L1 and L2

17. What nerve is involved in the clinical condition known as meralgia paresthetica?

Lateral femoral cutaneous nerve from L2 and L3

18. What are some of the typical causes of meralgia paresthetica?

Obesity. Weight loss. Clothing which is too constrictive at the proximal part of the thigh. Heavy pistol belt.

19. What spinal nerve levels are principally involved in the supply of the hamstring muscles?

Medial hamstrings: L5
Lateral hamstring (short head, biceps femoris): S1

20. What structures lie at the apex of the femoral triangle, from superficial to deep?

Femoral artery
Femoral vein
Deep femoral vein
Deep femoral artery

21. What nerve is damaged often in incisions or entrapped by scars at the medial side of the knee between the patella and the tibial tuberosity?

The infrapatellar branch of the saphenous nerve

LABORATORY IDENTIFICATION CHECK-LIST

The Thigh

surface features
great saphenous vein
saphenous   nerve

superficial circumflex iliac artery
superficial epigastric artery
superficial external pudendal artery

iliotibial tract

ilioinguinal nerve
lateral femoral cutaneous nerve
genitofemoral nerve
femoral nerve
obturator nerve

lumbosacral trunk

iliacus fascia, transversalis fascia
iliacus muscle

common iliac, internal iliac, external iliac artery
common iliac, internal iliac, external iliac vein
inferior epigastric artery and vein

origin of superior, inferior gluteal arteries
iliolumbar artery
lateral sacral artery
obturator artery

deep circumflex iliac artery and vein
femoral artery and vein
femoral sheath
femoral canal
femoral ring

lateral femoral cutaneous nerve of thigh
femoral nerve in thigh
sensory branches of femoral nerve in thigh

sartorius muscle
boundaries of femoral triangle
position, walls and extent of subsartorial canal
adductor hiatus
saphenous nerve in thigh, at origin, in canal
infrapatellar branch of the saphenous nerve

quadriceps tendon
rectus femoris, vastus medialis, vastus lateralis
vastus intermedius
nerves to quadriceps femoris muscle components
ligamentum patella

lateral femoral circumflex artery and vein;
    ascending, descending, and transverse branches
    of artery
nerve of the vastus medialis

profunda femoris artery and vein
medial femoral circumflex artery and vein

iliopsoas muscle and tendon
pectineus muscle
adductor longus muscle

perforating branches of profunda femoris
review components of cruciate anastomosis
gracilis muscle

anterior division of obturator nerve
adductor brevis muscle
posterior division of obturator nerve
adductor magnus muscle
hiatus of adductor magnus

obturator externus muscle
boundaries of subsartorial canal - review

DEFINITIONS

Calcaneus (pl. calcanei) - The irregular quadrangular bone at the back of the tarsus.

Fibula [L., "buckle"]
The outer and smaller of the two bones of the leg, which articulates proximally with the tibia and distally is joined to the tibia in a syndesmosis.

Linea aspera - A roughened longitudinal line with two lips, on the posterior surface of the shaft of the femur.

Malleolus (pl. malleoli) [L., dim. of *malleus,* hammer]
A rounded process, such as the protuberance on either side of the ankle joint.

Patella [L., dim. of *patera,* a shallow dish]
A triangular sesamoid bone, about five cm. in diameter, situated at the front of the knee in the tendon of insertion of the quadriceps extensor femoris muscle.

Profundus [L., deep]
A term denoting a structure situated deeper than another from the surface of the body.

Talus (pl. tali) [L., "ankle"]
The highest of the tarsal bones and the one which articulates with the tibia and fibula to form the ankle joint.

Tibia [L., "a pipe, flute"]
The shin bone: the inner and larger bone of the leg below the knee; it articulates with the femur and head of the fibula above and with the talus below.

CHAPTER 11

THE GLUTEAL REGION AND POSTERIOR THIGH

Review the osteology of the hipbone and femur, using figures 10:2, 3 in the previous chapter. Palpate the following structures upon yourself, a colleague, and the cadaver:

1. **Anterior superior iliac spine**
2. **Iliac crest**
3. **Posterior superior iliac spine**
4. **Greater trochanter**
5. **Ischial tuberosity**

*On a skeleton, identify the **greater** and **lesser** **sciatic** **notches**, **lesser** **trochanter**, **gluteal** **tuberosity**, **linea aspera** and features 1 - 5 above.*

The Iliotibial Tract and Lateral Intermuscular Septum. The iliotibial tract, as has been noted before, consists of thickened fascia lata, reinforced by the tendinous fibers of the tensor fasciae latae and gluteus maximus. The lateral intermuscular septum begins from the deep surface of the fascia lata and attaches to the linea aspera, thereby separating the extensor compartment from the flexor compartment of the thigh.

*With the cadaver in the supine position, place your fingers deep to the **iliotibial tract**, the band into which the **tensor fasciae latae muscle** and the **gluteus maximus muscle** (partially) insert. By digital exploration, observe the attachment of the **lateral intermuscular septum** to the linea aspera of the femur. With the fascia lata removed from the posterior surface of the thigh, it will be possible to feel the septum by inserting your fingers either anterior or posterior to the iliotibial tract. From an anterior approach, of course, your fingers will be inserted between the tract and the vastus lateralis.*

Superficial Dissection.

With the cadaver in the prone position, make an incision through the skin and subcutaneous tissues just inferior to the iliac crest, from the anterior superior iliac spine to the posterior superior iliac spine. [Note Figure 11:1.] Extend this incision medial to the cleft between the buttocks, veering away from the skin covering the perineum. Place an incision along the posterior aspect of the gluteal region and thigh, lateral to the midline of the limb. Finally, make a circumferential skin incision distal to the knee to limit the area of exposure. First, reflect the skin and then the superficial fascia from the gluteal region and thigh. Take special pains to identify the fascia lata of the posterior aspect of the thigh and leave it intact - to protect the posterior femoral cutaneous nerve, which lies just deep to this fascia in the midline posteriorly.

After the skin and superficial fascia have been removed from the gluteal region, posterior thigh and proximal part of the leg, make a small opening through the fascia lata of the thigh, near the midline

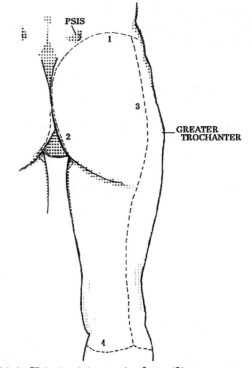

Figure 11:1 Skin incisions: 1, along iliac crest to PSIS (posterior superior iliac spine); 2, medially, around perineum; 3, down limb, posteriorly; 4, beyond knee, circumferentially.

178

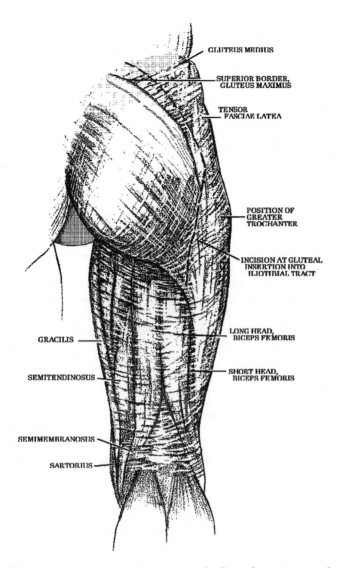

Figure 11:2 Posterior view of gluteal region and thigh, illustrating deep fascial and muscular relations. The broken line indicates the line of incision through the deep fascia and tendon of gluteus maximus.

*posteriorly, and find the **posterior femoral cutaneous nerve** (S1, 2, 3). Trace the nerve upward to its disappearance beneath the gluteus maximus. After the nerve and its branches have been cleaned this far, the fascia lata over the posterior compartment can be reflected and/or removed.*

The deep fascia surrounding the gluteus maximus joins at the superior border of this muscle and continues over the gluteus medius as the gluteal aponeurosis. This aponeurosis serves to obscure the plane of separation of the two muscles. Realize, however, that the muscular fibers of the gluteus medius run nearly perpendicular to the orientation of the gluteus maximus, and the two muscles can be readily separated once you have clearly exposed the fibers of the two muscles.

Clean all of the deep fascia from the surface of the gluteus maximus so that its superior and inferior borders can be delineated. Protect the posterior femoral cutaneous nerve from damage as the inferior border of the gluteus maximus is defined.

Cut through the deep fascia along the superior margin of the gluteus maximus, noting its relationship to the gluteus medius, as described above. Using your fingertips, lift the upper portion of the gluteus maximus from the underlying gluteus medius. Make a curving, nearly vertical incision through the tendinous portion of the gluteus maximus which inserts into the iliotibial tract (Fig.11:2).

The gluteus maximus has a broad origin from the ilium, sacrum, coccyx and ligamentous tissues of the area. Nearly three-fifths of this muscle inserts into the iliotibial tract; the remaining two-fifths inserts upon the gluteal tuberosity of the femur. The iliotibial tract inserts distally upon the lateral condyle of the tibia and is also anchored along the length of the femur by the lateral intermuscular septum. Thus, the power of the gluteus maximus acts to stabilize the knee joint, in addition to its action at the hip.

Where the tendinous deeper tissues of the gluteus maximus cross the greater trochanter, there is an intervening bursa lined with synovium, the **trochanteric bursa**. This bursa is frequently involved in disease processes. It functions normally, as do other bursae, to diminish the friction and wear and tear of tendinous fibers which pass over adjacent bony features. Pathology affecting bursae can result in erosion of the overlying tendons.

The gluteus maximus extends the hip joint for running, going up stairs, and arising from a seated or stooped position. It assists in maintaining upright posture, especially by its stabilizing actions at the knee joint. This muscle is innervated by the **inferior gluteal nerve** (L5, S1, S2).

*Bluntly reflect the gluteus maximus from the **greater trochanter** toward its origin medially and identify the **trochanteric bursa**.*

*Identify the **gluteus medius** and **tensor fasciae latae muscles** (Fig. 11:2, 3) clearly, removing enough of their deep fascial investments to expose the orientation of their muscular fibers and to clearly differentiate them from the gluteus maximus.*

*Reflect the gluteus maximus inferiorly and medially, sufficiently to begin to see the structures deep to it, including the **sciatic nerve**. The sciatic nerve passes just medial to the heavy, strong tendon of the gluteus maximus which inserts upon the **gluteal tuberosity** of the femur. Secure the sciatic nerve and the posterior femoral cutaneous nerve and protect them as you cut the tendon of the gluteus maximus away from the gluteal tuberosity. Continuing to protect the nerves, divide the deep fascia along the*

179

inferior border of the gluteus maximus, so that it can be reflected medially.

The **posterior femoral cutaneous nerve** (S1, 2, 3) is sensory to the posterior aspect of the extremity, from the lower border of the gluteus maximus (inferior cluneal branches) to a point just distal to the knee. In addition to providing sensory branches to the posterior and medial sides of the thigh, the posterior femoral cutaneous nerve also provides origin to one or more perineal branches.

The importance of the **perineal branch of the posterior femoral cutaneous nerve** lies in the fact that it provides some of the sensory supply to the tissues of the perineum and, in some women, it can provide the greater part of sensory fibers for the area - perhaps contributing to the difficulty with which anesthesia can be obtained for obstetric or surgical procedures.

*With the gluteus maximus fully reflected, identify and clean the **sciatic nerve** and the **posterior femoral cutaneous nerve** again, and trace them upward to their appearance from beneath the **piriformis muscle**. Identify the **perineal branch of the posterior femoral cutaneous nerve**. This nerve passes medially from the posterior femoral cutaneous nerve, under cover of the gluteus maximus, and then adjacent to the ischial tuberosity.*

*Upon a skeleton, again identify the **greater sciatic notch, spine of the ischium, ischial tuberosity** and the **lesser sciatic notch.***

The **sacrotuberous ligament** is attached proximally to the ilium, sacrum and coccyx; distally, it attaches to the tuberosity of the ischium. The gluteus maximus arises, in part, from the sacrotuberous ligament, as noted before. Deep to the sacrotuberous ligament, passing from the sacrum and coccyx to the spine of the ischium, is the **sacrospinous ligament**. By bridging the greater and lesser sciatic notches the sacrotuberous and sacrospinous ligaments convert the "notches" into the **greater** and **lesser sciatic foramina.**

*With careful use of the scalpel, reflect the gluteus maximus toward its origin to fully expose the **sacrotuberous ligament**. Divide the **inferior gluteal vessels** and **nerves**, as necessary, at their points of entrance into the muscle. Leave the gluteus maximus attached to the sacrum and upper, posterior parts of the ilium.*

*Clean the connective tissues from the structures which lie deep to the gluteus maximus. Fully expose the **piriformis muscle, inferior gluteal vessels** and **nerve**, the **sciatic nerve** and the **posterior femoral cutaneous nerve.***

The Gluteal "Door and Key". The greater sciatic foramen is usefully considered "the door" of the gluteal region for structures passing from the pelvis to the extremity, or vice versa. The lesser sciatic foramen forms a means of egress of the pudendal nerve and internal pudendal vessels - structures which enter the gluteal region through the greater sciatic foramen - but whose destination is the perineum.

The "key" to the gluteal region is the piriformis muscle. The piriformis arises **within** the pelvis from the anterior surface of the sacrum. The muscle passes through the greater sciatic foramen en route to its insertion upon the greater trochanter.

Certain structures enter the gluteal region by passing through the greater sciatic foramen and emerging either superior or inferior to the piriformis muscle.

The Suprapiriformic Space. The structures which enter the gluteal region superior to the piriformis (suprapiriformic space) are:
   (1) the superior gluteal nerve, and
   (2) the superior gluteal vessels. [The superior gluteal artery arises within the pelvis from the internal iliac artery - as was seen in the preceeding dissection.]

*Between the upper border of the piriformis and the gluteus medius muscle identify the **superficial branch of the superior gluteal artery and veins and the superior gluteal nerve.*** [As will be seen soon, the deep branch of the superior gluteal artery remains deep to the gluteus medius.]

The Infrapiriformic Space. Those structures that enter (or leave) the gluteal region by passing through the greater sciatic foramen **inferior** to the piriformis (infrapiriformic space) are:
   (1) the sciatic nerve;
   (2) the posterior femoral cutaneous nerve;
   (3) the inferior gluteal nerve;
   (4) the inferior gluteal artery and veins;
   (5) the internal pudendal artery and veins;
   (6) the pudendal nerve;
   (7) the nerve to the obturator internus, and
   (8) the nerve to the quadratus femoris.

Identify as many of the preceding structures as you can. The pudendal nerve, the internal pudendal vessels and the nerve to the obturator internus lie beneath the sacrotuberous ligament and will be sought in the connective tissue deep to the ligament, after identifying all of the muscles of the region. The nerve to the quadratus femoris can be found by dissecting carefully in the connective tissue deep to the sciatic nerve, just distal to the inferior border of the piriformis muscle.

Imagine a line drawn between the posterior superior iliac spine and the greater trochanter. Note that this line will pass rather close to, and parallel with, the piriformis muscle. Injections into the gluteal tissues should be placed well anterior to this line to avoid the sciatic nerve as it appears from

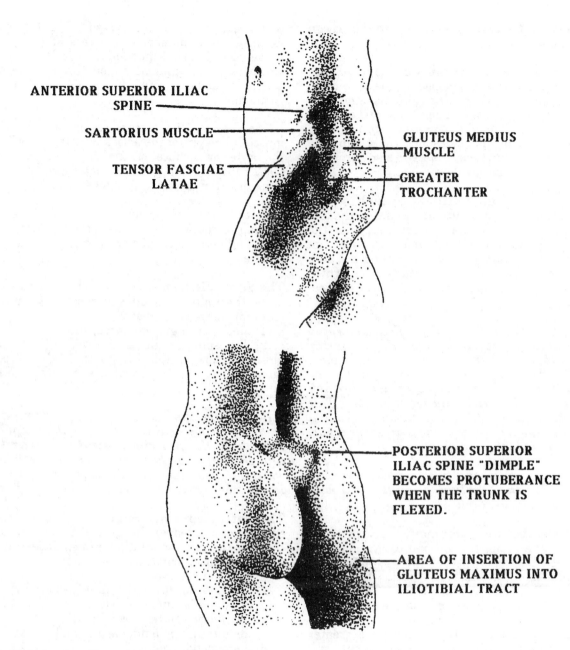

Figure 11:2 Surface Features of the gluteal region.

beneath the piriformis. In somewhat more than 10% of people part of the sciatic nerve penetrates the piriformis muscle, rather than emerging from beneath it. In such cases, the nerve is even more susceptible to trauma.

Thoughtless injections into the gluteal region can readily injure either the posterior femoral cutaneous nerve (with sensory loss), or more important, the sciatic nerve (which has extensive motor and sensory distribution), particularly in aged or thin individuals in whom the gluteal muscles are wasted and adipose tissue is scanty. Gluteal injections should, therefore, be confined to the superior lateral quadrant of the gluteal region.

The peroneal division of the sciatic nerve - the more lateral half or so of the nerve - is the more vulnerable portion and is damaged far more frequently than the medial, **tibial division**. Loss of the peroneal division results primarily in paralysis of dorsiflexor and evertor muscles of the foot, in addition to sensory loss on the dorsum of the foot.

The Obturator-Gemellus Complex. The **obturator internus muscle** arises **within** the pelvis from the internal surface of the hip bone and the obturator membrane, inferior to the true pelvic brim. From a somewhat triangularly-shaped field of origin, its muscle fibers converge to form a shiny white tendon which leaves the pelvis through the lesser sciatic foramen. The **superior and inferior gemelli** arise from the margins of the lesser sciatic

181

foramen, above and below the emerging obturator internus tendon. The three muscles combine as a tripartite muscle/tendon unit (referred to clinically as the "obturator-gemelli complex") which inserts upon the medial aspect of the greater trochanter. These muscles act syngergistically with other short lateral rotators of the hip joint.

Quadratus Femoris Muscle. The quadratus femoris muscle (not to be confused with the quadriceps femoris muscle) arises from the ischial tuberosity and inserts upon the proximal part of the femur, just below the intertrochanteric crest. This muscle, too, is a short lateral rotator of the hip joint. The quadratus femoris and the inferior gemellus are innervated by the nerve to the quadratus femoris.

Inferior to the piriformis muscle identify the **obturator internus muscle,** *the* **superior gemellus muscle** *and the* **inferior gemellus muscle.** *The obturator internus tendon and gemelli can be most readily separated at the margin of the lesser sciatic foramen.*

Inferior to the obturator internus and gemelli identify the **quadratus femoris.** *At the medial end of the quadratus identify the origins of the "hamstrings" (biceps femoris, semimembranosus, semitendinosus) from the ischial tuberosity. Deeply, and between the quadratus femoris and adductor magnus, identify the* **descending branch** *of the* **medial femoral circumflex artery.** *This vessel generally anastomoses with a branch of the inferior gluteal artery and the first perforating artery. The* **ascending branch of the medial circumflex artery** *passes superiorly, between the quadratus femoris and the obturator externus, to reach the neck of the femur, where it helps supply the hip joint. It can be seen if the quadratus femoris is cut from its insertion and reflected medially.*

Short Lateral Rotators of the Hip Joint. The piriformis, obturator internus, gemelli, the quadratus femoris and the obturator externus (which is not yet visible) insert in the region of the greater trochanter and are referred to collectively as the **short lateral rotators** of the thigh at the hip joint.

Deep to the sacrotuberous ligament identify - from lateral to medial - the **nerve to the obturator internus, internal pudendal artery** *and its* **venae comitantes** *and the* **pudendal nerve.** *These structures exit the pelvis through the greater sciatic foramen, cross the spine of the ischium and enter the perineum through the lesser sciatic foramen. Deep to these neural and vascular elements identify the* **sacrospinous ligament.** *The* **nerve to the obturator internus** *courses over the superior gemellus to supply it and then passes superficial to the obturator internus before passing through the lesser sciatc foramen.*

The Gluteus Medius and Gluteus Minimus Muscles. The gluteus medius is an extremely important abductor of the hip, arising broadly from the ilium and inserting upon the greater trochanter. Equally important is the fact that the gluteus medius muscle of one side of the body acts to keep the contralateral side of the pelvis from sagging when the limb of the contralateral side is lifted from the ground. [In other words, the functional origin and insertion can be reversed.] Loss of the gluteus medius causes one to lurch to the injured side, producing a pronounced limp which cannot be disguised, the so-called Trendelenberg sign.

Because muscle fibers arise from the ilium both anterior to, and posterior to, the position of the tip of the greater trochanter, the gluteus medius can also rotate the femur both medially and laterally at the hip joint.

The gluteus minimus arises from the ilium - although not so broad in its origin - deep to the gluteus medius, and inserts with the gluteus medius upon the greater trochanter. It acts to abduct and medially rotate the femur. Because its origin is situated more anteriorly, it is not particularly effective as a lateral rotator of the hip. Both the gluteus medius and gluteus minimus are supplied by the superior gluteal nerve (as is the tensor fasciae latae muscle).

Superior to the piriformis, identify the **gluteus medius** *muscle (Fig. 11:3) again. The* **superficial branch** *of the superior gluteal artery emerges between these two muscles to supply the upper portion of the gluteus maximus. Observe the regions of the ilium from which the gluteus medius and gluteus minimus arise.*

Reflect the gluteus medius anteriorly and inferiorly from its origin to see the **deep branch of the superior gluteal artery** *and the* **superior gluteal nerve** *on the deep surface of the gluteus medius. The nerve and artery lie within the plane of cleavage between the gluteus medius and the gluteus minimus. Identify the* **gluteus minimus** *muscle. Reflect the gluteus medius and gluteus minimus to their insertions upon the greater trochanter. [NOTE:* **The gluteus medius, minimus and tensor fasciae latae muscle are all innervated by the superior gluteal nerve** *from L4, 5, S1 - especially L5.]*

The Posterior Compartment of the Thigh

Note: *It is suggested that, while part of the dissection team explores the gluteal region, others proceed with the cleaning and identification of structures in the posterior compartment of the thigh.*

The muscles of the posterior, flexor chamber of the thigh include the semimembranosus, semitendinosus, the long head of the biceps femoris and the short head of the biceps femoris. The first three of these muscles, excluding the short head of the biceps femoris, are most often referred to as the "hamstrings." (Some include the short head of the biceps femoris in this designation.) The hamstring muscles have in common the facts that they arise from the ischial tuberosity, insert upon the bones of the leg, and act to flex the knee joint and extend the hip joint.

By blunt dissection, separate the muscles of the posterior chamber. Identify the **long head of the biceps femoris,** *the* **semitendinosus** *and the* **semimembranosus** *muscles. Clearly expose the origins of these, the "hamstrings", from the ischial tuberosity. Also identify the* **short head of the biceps femoris** *which originates from the linea aspera.*

Clean the **sciatic nerve,** *identifying its branches to the muscles of the flexor compartment and observing its division into the* **tibial** *and* **common peroneal nerves.** *The division of the sciatic nerve into the tibial and common peroneal nerves usually occurs near the knee; however, this separation may occur much earlier. Transect the long head of the biceps femoris and the semitendinosus distal to their innervation to better expose the sciatic nerve.*

The only muscle of the posterior chamber of the thigh innervated by the common peroneal portion (posterior divisions L4-S2) of the sciatic nerve is the **short head of the biceps femoris.** The short head of the biceps femoris arises from the linea aspera of the femur and the lateral intermuscular septum and joins the long head of the biceps femoris.

Identify the **nerve to the short head of the biceps femoris,** *the branch of the peroneal division of the sciatic nerve which supplies this muscle. Note that the nerve to the short head of the biceps is the only branch which arises from the lateral aspect of the sciatic nerve.*

Clean the **perforating arteries** *and* **veins** *which provide the arterial supply and venous drainage of the posterior compartment of the thigh. These perforating branches, as was discussed previously, originate from the deep femoral artery. The* **first perforating artery** *is commonly the largest of the series. You can usually find it proximally in the posterior compartment, just inferior to the insertion of the quadratus femoris, or as it pierces the adductor magnus, medial to the femoral insertion of the gluteus maximus.*

MUSCLES OF THE LOWER MEMBER
- A SUMMARY -

HIP AND GLUTEAL REGION

MUSCLE	ORIGIN	INSERTION	ACTIONS	INNERVATION
Gluteus maximus	Ilium, sacrum coccyx, ligaments of area	Gluteal tub. (2/5), iliotibial tract (3/5)	Extends and laterally rotates thigh; braces knee	Inferior gluteal nerve (L5, **S1**, S2)
Gluteus medius	Ilium	Greater trochanter	Abduction, rotation of thigh	Superior gluteal nerve (L4, **L5**, S1)
Gluteus minimus	Ilium	Greater trochanter	Abduction, medial rotation of thigh	Superior gluteal nerve (L4, **L5**, S1)
Tensor fasciae latae	Iliac crest; ant. superior spine	Iliotibial tract	Flexion of thigh	Superior gluteal nerve (L4, L5, S1)
Piriformis	Anterior surface of sacrum	Greater trochanter	Lateral rotator of thigh	Branch from sacral plexus
Obturator internus	Inner surface of bony pelvis	Greater trochanter	Lateral rotator of thigh	Nerve to obturator internus
Superior gemellus	Lesser sciatic notch	Greater trochanter	Lateral rotator of thigh	Nerve to obturator internus
Inferior gemellus	Lesser sciatic notch	Greater trochanter	Lateral rotator of thigh	Nerve to quadratus femoris
Quadratus femoris	Ischial tuberosity	Near greater trochanter	Lateral rotator and adductor of thigh	Nerve to quadratus femoris
Obturator externus	Outer surface of bony pelvis and obturator membrane	Trochanteric fossa	Lateral rotator of thigh	Obturator nerve
Iliopsoas	Iliac fossa; lumbar vertebrae	Lesser trochanter	Flexes thigh (or pelvis over thigh)	Lumbar nerves; femoral nerve (L1, L2)
Pectineus	Pectineal line of pubis	Pectineal line of femur	Flexes thigh, adducts thigh	Femoral nerve (or accessory obturator nerve)

QUESTIONS FOR REVIEW AND STUDY

1. What is the iliotibial tract?

It is an especially thickened portion of the fascia lata; it acts as a tendon of insertion for the tensor fasciae latae muscle and 3/5 of the gluteus maximus. The tract attaches to the lateral condyle of the tibia.

2. What are the functions of the gluteus maximus?

(a) By inserting upon the gluteal tuberosity of the femur-extension of the hip joint; (b) by inserting into the iliotibial tract- stabilizes the extended knee; (c) laterally rotates the thigh

3. Name the bones from which the gluteus maximus arises.

Ilium, sacrum, coccyx

4. What is the innervation of the gluteus maximus?

Inferior gluteal nerve.

5. What is the function of a bursa, in relation to tendon function?

Bursae, in somewhat of a lubricative fashion, allow tendons to move across bony protuberances without abrasion.

6. What arteries are severed as the upper border of the gluteus maximus is freed up?

Anastomosing branches of the superior gluteal, deep circumflex iliac and the ascending branch of the lateral femoral circumflex.

7. What is the source of cutaneous innervation to the buttocks?

Cluneal (gluteal) nerves: The superior cluneal nerves are lateral branches of DPR from upper lumbar (L1 - L3) nerves; the middle cluneal from DPR of sacral nerves (S1, S2, S3); inferior cluneal nerves are derived from the posterior femoral cutaneous nerve (S1, S2, S3).

8. What is the sensory supply to the posterior aspect of the thigh?

The posterior femoral cutaneous nerve.

9. What is the principal function of the tensor fasciae latae muscle?

Flexion of the thigh.

10. What is the motor supply of the tensor fasciae latae, gluteus minimus, gluteus medius?

The superior gluteal nerve.

11. Name two nerves that are of clincal significance when attempting anethesia of the perineum?

(1) The pudendal nerve
(2) Perineal branch of posterior femoral cutaneous nerve.

12. What structure separates the pudendal nerve and internal pudendal vessels from the gluteus maximus as they cross the ischial spine?

The sacrotuberous ligament.

13. What is the "key" to the gluteal region? What is its clinical significance?

The piriformis muscle. To avoid damage to the sciatic nerve, injections should be made superior and lateral to the position of this muscle.

14. What is the "door" to the gluteal region and why is it called this?

The greater sciatic foramen is the "door" of the gluteal region, because it provides a passageway for nerves and vessels between the pelvis and gluteal region.

15. Name the structures
    a. that appear inferior to the piriformis muscle in the gluteal region.

a. Inferior gluteal artery, veins, nerve; posterior femoral cutaneous nerve; sciatic nerve; pudendal nerve; internal pudendal artery and veins; nerve to obturator internus.

    b. which appear superior to this muscle.

b. Superior gluteal artery (superficial branch), veins, nerve.

16. Name the short lateral rotators of the thigh.

Piriformis, obturator externus, the two gemelli, quadratus femoris, and the obturator internus.

17. Name the hamstring muscles.

Biceps femoris, semitendinosus and semimembranosus. Each of these arises at the ischial tuberosity and passes to insertion at the knee, without attaching to the femur (except for the short head of the biceps femoris).

18. What is the origin of the sciatic nerve?

L4, 5; S1, 2, 3

19. What is the origin of the superior gluteal nerve, with respect to spinal cord levels?

L4, 5, S1

20. What is the origin of the inferior gluteal nerve, with respect to spinal cord levels?

L5, S1, 2

21. What other muscle is innervated by the nerve to the obturator internus?

The superior gemellus

22. What other muscle is innervated by the nerve to the quadratus femoris?

The inferior gemellus

23. What artery passes between the gluteus medius and gluteus minimus?

The deep branch of the superior gluteal artery.

24. How does the lower extremity receive sympathetic supply (for innervation of sweat glands, pilomotor muscles and blood vessels)?

Preganglionic sympathetic neurons in upper lumbar segments of IML; white rami at L1, L2, preganglionic fibers descend in sympathetic chain to gray rami at lower lumbar and sacral levels; into ventral rami of lumbar and sacral plexuses; distributed to lower limb.

25. What is the function of the gluteus medius?

This muscle abducts and rotates the hip medially and laterally. It acts to tilt the pelvis over the ipsilateral limb, or to keep the contralateral side of the pelvis from sagging when the opposite limb is lifted from the ground.

LABORATORY IDENTIFICATION CHECK-LIST

The Gluteal Region

REVIEW:

anterior superior iliac spine
posterior superior iliac spine
pubic tubercles
symphysis pubis
greater trochanter, lesser trochanter
medial, lateral femoral condyles
tibial tuberosity
head of the fibula
medial, lateral malleoli of ankle
great saphenous vein
saphenous nerve

saphenous hiatus
cribriform fascia
superficial inguinal lymph nodes
superficial tributaries to great saphenous vein
fascia lata
iliotibial tract
tensor fasciae latae muscle
gluteus maximus muscle
lateral intermuscular septum of thigh
linea aspera

gluteal tuberosity of femur
gluteus medius muscle
trochanteric bursa
sciatic nerve
posterior femoral cutaneous nerve
perineal branch of posterior femoral cutaneous nerve
sacrotuberous ligament

piriformis muscle
inferior gluteal artery, vein
inferior gluteal nerve
greater sciatic notch
lesser sciatic notch

tuberosity of ischium
sacrospinous ligament
greater and lesser sciatic foramina
obturator internus muscle
superior and inferior gemellus muscles
quadratus femoris muscle
common origin of hamstrings
nerve to obturator internus
internal pudendal artery and venae comites
pudendal nerve
gluteus minimus muscle
superior gluteal artery (superficial and deep branches) and venae comites
superior gluteal nerve
medial femoral circumflex artery and venae comites

long head of biceps femoris muscle
semitendinosus muscle
semimembranosus muscle
short head of biceps femoris muscle

nerve to short head of biceps

peroneal division of sciatic nerve
tibial division of sciatic nerve
nerve supply of hamstring muscles

perforating branches of profunda femoris artery
perforating tributaries to profunda femoris vein

DEFINITIONS

Cluneal [L. *clunis*, the buttock]

Gluteal [Gr. *gloutos*, the buttock]

Perineum [Gr. *peri*, around + *neos*, young or new, newborn]
The meaning of this term is somewhat obscure in its origin, although it may translate to mean the region surrounding the outlet for childbirth

Piriformis [L. *pirum*, a pear, pear-shaped]

Obturator [L. *obturare*, to stop up or occlude]
The obturator foramen of the bony pelvis is almost entirely closed over by the obturator membrane and the obturator muscles.

Trochanter [Gr. *trokanter*, a roller, or runner]
This term was applied originally to the head of the femur, but was later applied to processes which acted like levers for the rotary movments of the thigh.

CHAPTER 12

THE LEG

*Using Figure 12:1 and skeletal material, study the principal bony features of the leg. Palpate the **head of the fibula,** the **tibial condyles,** the **tuberosity and anterior border of the tibia,** the **lateral malleolus** and the **medial malleolus.** Palpate these features upon yourself and then the cadaver.*

With your knee flexed, attempt to palpate the tendons which attach about the level of the knee (Fig. 12:2). Laterally, identify the tendon of insertion of the iliotibial tract and, posterior to it, the tendon of the biceps femoris. Medially, palpate the tendon of the semimembranosus. This tendon inserts upon the posterior surface of the tibia. Medially and somewhat more superficially, identify the tendon of the semitendinosus. The semitendinosus tendon joins the tendons of the sartorius and gracilis, inserting upon the medial aspect of the proximal part of the tibia.

Superficial Dissection

Great Saphenous Vein, Saphenous Nerve. The saphenous nerve accompanies the great saphenous vein in their course inferior to the knee, from the medial malleolus to the medial femoral condyle, and provides sensory supply to the anterior and medial aspect of the leg and the medial side of the foot and great toe. The saphenous nerve is the longest sensory branch of the femoral nerve.

*Remove the skin from the leg to the level of the malleoli. Take pains to leave the superficial and deep fascia (crural fascia) intact to protect underlying structures. Review the origin, course and termination of the **great saphenous vein.** Identify the **saphenous nerve** again.*

Small Saphenous Vein, Sural Nerve. The small (lesser) saphenous vein arises from the lateral aspect of the dorsal venous arch of the foot, passes up the posterior aspect of the leg and terminates in the popliteal vein within the popliteal fossa. The small

saphenous vein often has large anastomoses with the great saphenous vein near the knee, after which the lesser saphenous vein may be quite small. It also may end by joining the profunda femoris vein or one of its tributaries.

The **sural nerve** is formed by the combination of a **medial sural cutaneous nerve** (from the tibial nerve) and the **communicating branch of the lateral sural cutaneous nerve.** The medial sural cutaneous nerve is often hidden proximally by overlying tendinous fibers of the gastrocnemius. The medial and lateral sural cutaneous nerves are sensory to the posterior and lateral aspects of the leg. The sural nerve distributes cutaneous branches to the posterior surface of the distal portion of the leg, then passes beneath the lateral malleolus. In the foot the sural nerve becomes the **lateral dorsal cutaneous nerve,** supplying the lateral side of the foot and the fifth toe.

*In the superficial fascia upon the posterior aspect of the leg identify the **small,** or lesser, **saphenous vein.** Clean and preserve the nerve which accompanies the short saphenous vein, the sural nerve. Look for the communicating branch of the lateral sural cutaneous nerve at its junction with the medial sural cutaneous nerve to form the sural nerve.*

*Trace the **communicating branch of the lateral sural cutaneous nerve** upward toward the popliteal fossa to expose its origin from the lateral sural cutaneous nerve. The lateral sural cutaneous nerve is a branch of the common peroneal nerve. Use scissors to cut the tendinous fibers of the gastrocnemius which cover the **medial sural cutaneous nerve** and expose the nerve to its origin from the tibial nerve.*

Trace the small saphenous vein into the popliteal fossa. Note its tributaries from superficial and deep perforating veins. Look for a direct communication between the great and short saphenous veins near the knee and note its manner of termination.

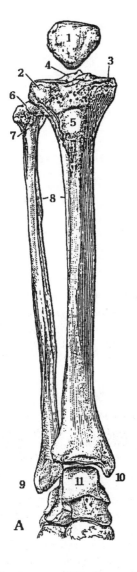
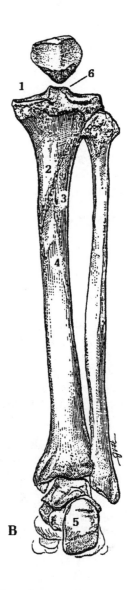

Figure 12:1 The bones of the leg and ankle. A, Anterior view; B, Posterior view.

1. Patella
2. Lateral condyle of tibia
3. Medial condyle of tibia
4. Intercondylar eminence
5. Tibial tuberosity
6. Head of fibula
7. Neck of fibula
8. Interosseous borders of shafts of tibia and fibula
9. Lateral malleolus
10. Medial malleolus
11. Articular surface of talus

1. Tibial plateau
2. Soleal (popliteal) line
3. Nutrient canal of tibia
4. Shaft (body) of tibia
5. Calcaneal tuberosity
6. Intercondylar eminence

Superficial Peroneal Nerve. A third sensory nerve of importance makes its appearance from the deep fascia in the distal third of the anterolateral aspect of the leg, the **superficial peroneal nerve** (musculocutaneous nerve). The superficial peroneal nerve innervates the muscles of the lateral chamber of the leg (peroneus longus, peroneus brevis) and then emerges through the deep fascia to provide much of

the sensory supply to the dorsum of the foot (L5 dermatome) and digits. The superficial peroneal nerve arises from the common peroneal nerve (near the neck of the fibula) after the common peroneal nerve has entered the lateral muscular compartment of the leg.

The superficial peroneal nerve lies in a position which is rather vulnerable to lacerations of the lower, lateral surface of the leg or ankle. Its presence must be kept in mind also by surgeons who must make incisions in the skin near its emergence, or its course. You can readily see, for instance, that if one were to make an incision to expose the fibula for repair, or

190

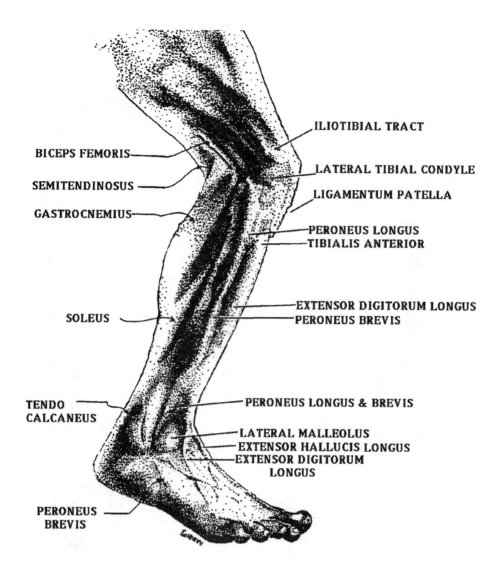

BICEPS FEMORIS

SEMITENDINOSUS

GASTROCNEMIUS

SOLEUS

TENDO
CALCANEUS

PERONEUS
BREVIS

ILIOTIBIAL TRACT

LATERAL TIBIAL CONDYLE

LIGAMENTUM PATELLA

PERONEUS LONGUS
TIBIALIS ANTERIOR

EXTENSOR DIGITORUM LONGUS
PERONEUS BREVIS

PERONEUS LONGUS & BREVIS

LATERAL MALLEOLUS
EXTENSOR HALLUCIS LONGUS
EXTENSOR DIGITORUM
LONGUS

Figure 12:2 Surface features of the lateral aspect of the leg.

for other reasons, the superficial peroneal nerve could be inadvertently severed, particularly if its presence were unsuspected.

Compartmentalization of the Leg. The leg is surrounded by a stout layer of deep fascia, the **crural fascia**. This fascia, plus the bones, an interosseous membrane, and intermuscular septae separate and enclose three muscular compartments, each of which has its own source of innervation (Fig. 12:3).

The **anterior,** or **extensor, compartment** contains three muscles which act to dorsiflex the foot at the ankle, invert the foot, and extend the toes. They receive their nerve supply from the deep peroneal nerve, a branch of the common peroneal nerve. The anterior compartment is bounded medially by the tibia, posteriorly by the interosseous membrane and laterally by the **anterior intermuscular septum**, a longitudinal band which arises from the deep fascia and attaches to the fibula.

The **lateral,** or **evertor, compartment** contains two muscles which arise from the fibula and function to evert the foot. These are supplied by the superficial peroneal nerve.

The muscles of the **posterior,** or **flexor, compartment** are separated from the other compartments by the tibia, interosseous membrane and the posterior intermuscular septum. This compartment is subdivided further by a fascial plane into superficial, intermediate and deep subcompartments.

The compartmentalization of the leg by relatively unyielding bony and fascial boundaries is clinically important, especially in the causation and treatment of compartmental compression syndromes. For example, severe blunt trauma to the front of the leg can in some cases result in the **five signs of elevated intracompartmental pressure** from

191

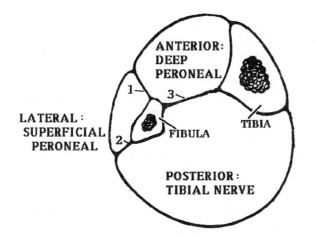

Figure 12:3 Schematic cross section, illustrating the compartmentalization and nerve supply of the leg. 1, Anterior intermuscular septum; 2, posterior intermuscular septum; 3, interosseous membrane.

bleeding or edema: **p**ain, **p**allor, **p**uffiness, **p**aresthesia and **p**aralysis. Leakage of small vessels first leads to an elevation of interstitial pressure. If this pressure increases sufficiently, venous drainage can become occluded. Should this occur, continued arterial inflow causes the pressure to escalate even more rapidly. Finally, the internal pressure becomes so great as to restrict, or cut off, arterial supply altogether. Ischemic necrosis of tissues can then take place rapidly.

Muscles can withstand six to eight hours of ischemia, but nerves can tolerate only about two hours of deficiency of vascular supply. Necrosis of musculature is followed often by its replacement by fibrous tissue, causing shortening of the tissue mass and contracture of the affected limb parts. This is known clinically as **Volkmann's ischemic contracture.**

Other causes of compartmental pressure syndromes include unaccustomed muscular overexertion, snakebite, infection, fractures and injection of foreign toxic materials (such as paint or grease from compressed-air equipment).

One common means of treating compartmental compression problems is the use of **fasciotomy,** wherein a wide incision is made in the deep fascia. This allows the tissues to swell with less restriction of vascular supply. In practice, the wound can be left open, covered with a sterile dressing, until the swelling subsides and then the wound can be closed. In certain cases, such as in injection of toxic foreign material into a compartment, the separate sheaths of muscles within the compartment may also require separate fasciotomies.

The Sciatic Nerve. The sciatic nerve, as has been seen already, divides into the **tibial** and **common peroneal nerves.** The tibial (posterior tibial) nerve supplies motor branches to all of the muscles of the posterior chamber of the leg (flexor compartment) and then divides at the ankle into the medial and lateral plantar nerves, which provide motor and sensory supply to the sole of the foot.

The common peroneal nerve passes anteriorly around the neck of the fibula into the lateral compartment of the leg (peroneal compartment) and then divides into **superficial** and **deep** (anterior tibial) **peroneal nerves** within the proximal part of the peroneus longus. The superficial peroneal nerve innervates the muscles of the lateral (evertor) compartment and then continues as a cutaneous nerve as discussed above. The deep peroneal nerve supplies the anterior (extensor) compartment of the leg and short muscles on the dorsum of the foot and ends as a sensory nerve between the first and second toes.

The Popliteal Fossa

The Boundaries of the Popliteal Fossa. The popliteal fossa is the roughly diamond - or rhomboid - shaped region posterior to the knee joint. Its boundaries are:
   (1) superolateral - the biceps femoris;
   (2) superomedial - the tendons of the semitendinosus and semimembranosus;
   (3) inferolateral - lateral head of the gastrocnemius;
   (4) inferomedial - the medial head of the gastrocnemius.

The Contents of the Fossa. Upon, or within, the popliteal fossa are:
   (1) the **posterior femoral cutaneous nerve;**
   (2) the **small, or lesser, saphenous vein;**
   (3) the **tibial and common peroneal nerves;**
   (4) the **popliteal vein and its tributaries;**
   (5) the **popliteal artery and its branches;**
   (6) several **lymph nodes;**
   (7) adipose and areolar tissue.

The **floor** of the popliteal fossa is provided by the distal end of the femur, the capsule of the knee joint and the popliteus muscle (to be exposed later).

Clean the fascia, adipose tissue and lymph nodes from the popliteal fossa and inspect the boundaries of the region. Identify as many of the above listed structures as possible, while cleaning away the adipose and areolar tissue.

Vascular Supply. The femoral artery becomes the **popliteal artery** at its passage through the hiatus of the adductor magnus. The popliteal artery terminates by dividing into the **anterior** and **posterior tibial arteries** just inferior to the popliteus muscle. Arising from the popliteal artery are **superolateral, superomedial, inferolateral, inferomedial** and **middle genicular arteries.**

The genicular branches of the popliteal artery, the descending branch of the lateral femoral circumflex, the supreme genicular branch of the femoral artery and recurrent branches of the tibial arteries participate in anastomoses about the knee. The anastomoses about the knee are very important in slowly progressing vascular occlusive diseases; however, sudden occlusion of the popliteal artery leads frequently to gangrene of the leg. The **popliteal vein** is formed by the junction of the venae comitantes of the tibial arteries.

Note the relationships of the large vessels which have been studied in the limb:
(1) at the inguinal ligament the femoral artery is **lateral** to the vein;
(2) at the apex of the femoral triangle the femoral artery is **anterior** and **superficial** to the femoral vein;
(3) in the popliteal fossa, the popliteal vein is **superficial,** but **posterior,** to the artery. In the popliteal fossa the two great vessels are so intimately juxtaposed that penetrating injuries can readily lead, in time, to arteriovenous fistulas.

The Posterior Compartment of the Leg.

Crural Fascia. The **crural fascia**, the deep fascia of the leg, is quite dense and forms a stocking-like investment about the member, which is continuous with the fascia lata of the thigh. Due to its investment of superficial veins and its attachments to underlying muscles, crural fascia is important in assisting the normal venous and lymphatic return from the extremity.

Contents. The muscles of the posterior chamber can be placed into groups for convenience of study as follows.
(1) Superficial: gastrocnemius, plantaris, soleus;
(2) Middle, or intermediate: popliteus, flexor digitorum longus, flexor hallucis longus;
(3) Deep: tibialis posterior.

The Gastrocnemius, Soleus and Plantaris Muscles. The **medial and lateral heads of the gastrocnemius** arise from the femoral condyles and the capsule of the knee joint. The two heads fuse distally, and are joined by the deeper, soleus muscle to form the so-called **triceps surae muscle** (the three-headed muscle of the calf). The **soleus** arises by broad attachments to the tibia and fibula.

By a common tendon, the achilles tendon, or **tendo calcaneus**, the gastrocnemius and soleus muscles insert upon the calcaneus bone of the foot. The triceps surae muscle is the most powerful plantar flexor of the foot at the ankle joint and help to maintain balance. In addition, because of the femoral origin of the two heads of the gastrocnemius muscle, the gastrocnemius muscle assists in flexion of the knee. The gastrocnemius and soleus muscles are supplied by the tibial nerve.

The **plantaris** arises above the lateral condyle of the femur, but its tendon passes diagonally to the medial aspect of the soleus. This slender tendon, frequently referred to as the "freshman's nerve," inserts upon the medial aspect of the **calcaneus bone** of the foot or upon the medial aspect of the **tendo calcaneus.**

*Remove all of the deep fascia from the posterior chamber of the leg, baring the muscles, if this has not already been done. Identify the **medial** and **lateral** heads of the gastrocnemius muscle and trace their innervation from the tibial nerve, and their arterial supply from the popliteal artery. Secure the **common peroneal nerve** and trace it to the neck of the fibula. Again, identify and preserve its **lateral sural cutaneous** branch.*

*Note the **medial sural cutaneous** branch of the tibial nerve and move it aside, then incise each head of the gastrocnemius distal to its innervation. Reflect the gastrocnemius muscle inferiorly, preserving the nerves and vessels of the region. Identify the **soleus muscle** and the long, slender tendon of the **plantaris muscle.***

*Attempt to identify the **nerve to the soleus** from the tibial nerve. Sever the attachment of the soleus from the upper third of the fibula. Taking precautions to protect the tibial nerve and adjacent vessels, divide the origin of the soleus at the tibia, then reflect the soleus and gastrocnemius together toward the ankle to expose the deeper muscles.*

*The **superolateral and superomedial genicular arteries** are most readily found by carefully scraping aside the fat and connective tissue covering the femur just above the origins of the lateral and medial heads of the gastrocnemius, respectively. Do not be misled by muscular branches of the popliteal artery. The genicular branches arise from the popliteal artery and pass deeply toward the level of the bony femur quite early in their courses. The **middle genicular artery** should be sought at its origin from the deep surface of the popliteal artery, passing directly forward (anterior) into the knee joint.*

*The **inferolateral genicular artery** can be identified if you will first lift the lateral head of the gastrocnemius muscle and look deep to it. The artery crosses the <u>origin</u> of the popliteus muscle and can be seen if you clear away the connective tissue covering the muscle. At a similar depth medially, beneath the medial head of the gastrocnemius, you can find the **inferomedial genicular artery** where it courses along the cranial border of the popliteus muscle.*

The Popliteus, Flexor Hallucis Longus and Flexor Digitorum Longus Muscles. According to most anatomy textbooks, the short, quadrilateral **popliteus** muscle arises from the lateral condyle of the femur, within the fibrous capsule of the knee joint, and passes obliquely downward in a medial direction to the tibia. Functionally, however, one should probably say that the muscle arises from the posterior side of the tibia and inserts upon the lateral condyle of the femur - thereby reversing the origin and insertion of the muscle as typically stated. In its principal action, the popliteus rotates the femur laterally on the tibia when the foot is planted and the knee is in full extension. Thus it "unlocks" the knee from extension and assists in knee flexion.

The **flexor hallucis longus** arises from the fibula, thereby gaining additional mechanical advantage, as its tendon exits from the **medial** aspect of the leg into the foot - and inserts upon the plantar surface of the distal phalanx of the great toe. The **flexor digitorum longus** arises from the tibia and inserts into the distal phalanges of the other digits. Both muscles produce plantar (toward the ground) flexion of the toes and foot.

The Tibialis Posterior Muscle. The tibialis posterior arises from the posterior surface of the interosseous membrane, tibia and fibula to insertion principally upon the navicular bone and first cuneiform bone in the foot. This muscle flexes and inverts the foot (turns the sole inward) and provides strong support to the longitudinal arch of the foot.

*Identify the **popliteus muscle** and its **nerve**. The dense fibrous tissue which covers the muscle may make it somewhat difficult to see initially. The nerve to the popliteus muscle runs parallel with the anterior tibial artery, entering the inferior border of the popliteus muscle. Separate the **flexor hallucis longus** and **flexor digitorum longus**. To identify the deepest muscle of the compartment, the **tibialis posterior**, first trace out the arteries of the posterior compartment.*

Arteries of the Posterior Compartment. The popliteal artery usually divides into anterior and posterior tibial arteries near the lower border of the popliteus muscle. The **anterior tibial** arises from the anterior, or deep, surface of the popliteal artery and courses over, or through, a gap in the interosseous membrane into the anterior chamber of the leg. The **posterior tibial artery**, the other terminal branch of the popliteal, passes inferiorly and gives origin to a **peroneal branch** which passes deep to the flexor hallucis longus, providing a plane of cleavage between the flexor hallucis longus and the underlying tibialis posterior muscle.

*Clean the **posterior tibial artery**, veins and tibial nerve to the level of the ankle. Identify and clean the **peroneal branch of the posterior tibial artery**. If the peroneal artery is followed and cleaned, you will find the plane of cleavage between the flexor hallucis longus and the more deeply situated tibialis posterior. The tendons of these muscles are more easily separated for identification near the ankle.*

Lateral Compartment

The Peroneus Longus and Peroneus Brevis Muscles. Common Peroneal Nerve. The lateral compartment contains two muscles, together with their neural and vascular supply. The two muscles are the peroneus longus and peroneus brevis.

The **peroneus longus** arises from the proximal portion, the peroneus brevis - situated more deeply - from the distal aspect of the lateral surface of the fibula. The tendons of the two muscles pass posterior to the lateral malleolus and then turn obliquely forward. The **peroneus brevis** inserts upon the fifth metatarsal bone (posterior to the insertion of the peroneus tertius). The peroneus longus passes about the lateral aspect of the foot into the sole, inserting medially upon the first cuneiform and first metatarsal. Both the peroneus longus and the peroneus brevis are evertors of the foot.

The **common peroneal nerve** lies just posterior to the tendon of the biceps femoris until reaching the level of the fibular neck. Winding anteriorly around the neck of the fibula, the common peroneal nerve enters the substance of the peroneus longus and immediately divides into the superficial peroneal nerve and the deep peroneal nerve.

The **superficial peroneal nerve** supplies the peroneus longus and the peroneus brevis; then, continuing its course inferiorly along the anterior intermuscular septum, it pierces the deep fascia to emerge as a cutaneous nerve. The **deep peroneal nerve** passes through the anterior intermuscular septum to reach the anterior compartment of the leg, which it supplies, thereafter passing to the dorsum of the foot.

*Divide the crural fascia covering the lateral, or peroneal, compartment of the leg and separate the two muscles of this compartment - the **peroneus longus and brevis**. [Remember that, despite the similarity in names, the peroneus tertius is **not** a muscle of the lateral compartment.]*

*Trace the common peroneal nerve about the fibula into the lateral chamber. Excise enough of the peroneus longus to identify the bifurcation of the common peroneal into the **deep peroneal nerve** (motor to the anterior chamber) and the **superficial peroneal nerve** (or, **musculocutaneous nerve**), which is motor to the lateral compartment). Trace the superficial sensory portion of the superficial peroneal nerve to its passage distally from the lateral compartment to the dorsum of the foot - to which it is the principal source of sensory supply.*

Anterior Compartment

The Tibialis Anterior, Extensor Hallucis Longus, Extensor Digitorum Longus and Peroneus Tertius Muscles. The tibialis anterior arises from a long strip along the lateral surface of

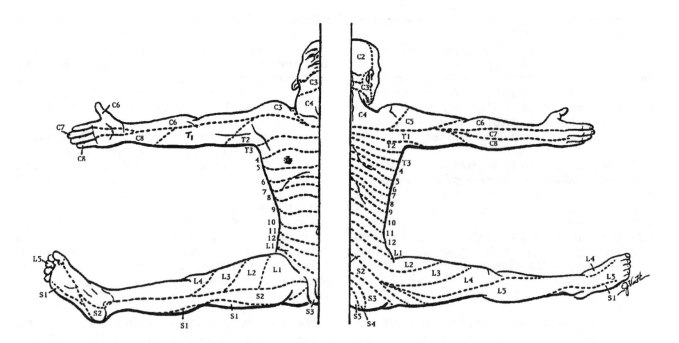

Figure 12:4 Dermatome distribution in the lower limb, as seen from ventral and dorsal points of view.

the tibia.   The tendon of the **tibialis anterior** appears proximally between the tibia and the extensor digitorum longus and then passes distally in front of the medial malleolus toward its insertion upon the first cuneiform and first metatarsal. Like the tibialis posterior, the tibialis anterior inverts the foot, but it also dorsiflexes the foot.

The **extensor hallucis longus** emerges in the distal one-third of the extensor compartment between the tibialis anterior and the extensor digitorum longus. The tendon of the extensor hallucis longus inserts at the base of the distal phalanx of the great toe for extension of that digit. It also dorsiflexes the foot. The **extensor digitorum longus** arises primarily from the fibula and distributes tendons to the lateral four toes. Like the extensor hallucis, this muscle also dorsiflexes the foot, in addition to toe extension.

Distal to the extensor digitorum longus, a small muscle diverges laterally from the extensor digitorum muscle and passes to insertion on the base of the fifth metatarsal bone. This muscle is named separately as the **peroneus tertius.** The peroneus tertius assists both in dorsiflexion and **eversion** of the foot (turning the sole outwards.) The principal evertors of the foot are, of course, situated in the lateral compartment.

Each of the four muscles of the anterior compartment of the leg receives its motor nerve supply from the deep peroneal nerve.

*Place the body in the supine position, if necessary. Make a longitudinal incision through the crural fascia one inch lateral to the subcutaneous portion of the tibia, from the level of the tuberosity of the tibia to the level of the malleoli. Keeping the fascia as intact as possible, reflect it laterally to expose the muscles of the anterior (extensor) compartment. Identify the **anterior intermuscular septum** which separates the anterior and lateral muscular compartments. Identify the muscles of the anterior compartment - the **tibialis anterior, extensor digitorum longus, extensor hallucis longus** and **peroneus tertius.***

*Between the tibialis anterior and the extensor digitorum longus identify and clean the **anterior tibial artery** and the **deep peroneal nerve** (anterior tibial nerve), one of the terminal branches of the common peroneal nerve.   Trace the anterior tibial artery proximally until it is clearly observed passing above the proximal end or through the interosseous membrane.   Trace the deep peroneal nerve to its entrance into the anterior chamber.*

Neurologic Aspects of the Lower Limb. The most common source of the neurologic problems in the lower limb is vertebral disk herniation, or other causes of compression or damage to the lumbar and sacral spinal nerve roots.   In the   upper limb, lacerations or trauma to peripheral nerves or their branches are more common than injuries to the spinal nerve roots of the limb.

195

Injuries to peripheral nerves in the lower limb occur far less frequently than to those in the upper limb. Also, in generalizing, one can note that in the lower limb the muscles are more massive and tend to be supplied by two or more spinal nerve levels, with less tendency toward the relationship seen more in the upper limb of a single, dominant spinal nerve supply for a specific muscle or muscle group. There are several muscles or muscle groups in the lower limb, however, for which a single spinal nerve level is most significant in innervation; such lend themselves to clinical evaluation and discrimination between spinal nerve root and peripheral nerve lesion.

Sensory Distribution of Spinal Nerves. Review the dermatome distribution pattern in the lower limb shown in Figure 12:4. Note in particular the following few useful facts regarding spinal nerve supply of sensory fibers to the limb - which hold true for a large portion of the human population:

L4 - The medial aspect of the leg and foot. L4 is also the most important nerve root level in carrying the afferent limb of the patellar reflex arc.

L5 - The lateral aspect of the leg, the dorsum of the foot and the sole of the foot.

S1 - Distribution is most significant in the supply of a strip of skin down the posterior aspect of the thigh, the leg, and the lateral aspect of the foot. S1 also carries the afferent limb of the Achilles reflex (ankle jerk).

Motor Distribution of Spinal Nerves. There is a generalized proximal to distal distribution of spinal nerve supply to the muscles of the lower limb; for instance:

L1, 2 - Hip flexors
L2, 3 - Knee extensors and thigh adductors
L4 - Foot invertors, especially tibialis anterior and posterior
L4, 5 - Dorsiflexors and extensors of the foot
L5 - Extension of the great toe
S1 - Hip extension, but also plantar flexion of foot, eversion of foot
S2 - Toe push-off muscles
S2, 3 - Intrinsic muscles of the sole of the foot

An isolated lesion of the **fourth lumbar spinal nerve** can often be associated with the following clinical signs (in synthesizing the data given above): Pain or anesthesia of the medial aspect of the leg and foot; a lessening of the patellar reflex, with little reduction in the strength of knee extension; weakness in inversion of the foot. Note that foot inversion involves two muscles particularly, the tibialis anterior and the tibialis posterior - muscles which are in different compartments and supplied by different peripheral nerves. One receives its L4 fibers from the anterior division of the ventral primary ramus, and the other receives fibers from the posterior division.

A lesion of the **fifth lumbar spinal nerve** will, in many patients, result in weakness of dorsiflexion of the foot, and particular weakness in the extensor hallucis longus. Sensory problems can involve both the dorsum and the sole of the foot and, peculiarly, pain in the great toe.

Problems of the **first sacral spinal nerve** occur very often. In the person affected, there may be a line of pain down the posterior aspect of the limb which passes to the lateral side of the foot. Weakness in eversion of the foot is common, and some weakness may occur in plantar flexion, with reduction or loss of the Achilles tendon reflex.

Peripheral Nerve Lesions in the Lower Limb. As noted above, lesions of the peripheral nerves of the lower limb occur less frequently than they do in the upper limb. The peroneal division of the sciatic nerve (or the common peroneal nerve) is, by far, the most commonly injured. It is subject to trauma in the gluteal region from perforating injuries or injections - as noted in the study of the gluteal area. It is very readily damaged in the vicinity of the knee, especially as it passes about the neck of the fibula.

Injury of the common peroneal nerve results in "foot drop", wherein the patient cannot dorsiflex nor evert the foot, with accompanying sensory deficits, as well. Damage can be induced at the knee from diverse causes such as blunt trauma, compression from pressure applied by a cast, resting the patient's leg on a sandbag during some other related or unrelated treatment, and so on.

The preceding facts can assist one in developing an appreciation for the importance of precise information when trying to understand a patient's signs and symptoms, especially when trying to decide whether those signs and symptoms indicate the presence of a spinal nerve root problem or dysfunction of a peripheral nerve.

TABLE 12:1 MUSCLES OF THE LOWER MEMBER
- A SUMMARY -

THE LEG

MUSCLE	ORIGIN	INSERTION	FUNCTION	INNERVATION
Gastrocnemius	Medial, lateral femoral condyles	Calcaneus	Flexes knee; plantar flexes foot	Tibial nerve (S1, 2)
Soleus	Upper third, fibula; middle third, tibia	Calcaneus	Plantar flexes foot	Tibial nerve (S1, 2)
Plantaris	Distal lateral linea aspera	Calcaneus	Flexes knee, weakly plantar flexes foot	Tibial nerve (L4, 5, S1)
Popliteus	Lateral condyle of femur	Popliteal line of tibia	Flexes knee, rotates leg medially	Tibial nerve (L4, 5, S1)
Flexor Hallucis Longus	Inferior 2/3 of fibula	Distal phalanx of hallux	Flexes hallux; plantar flexes and inverts foot	Tibial nerve (L5, S1, 2)
Flexor Digitorum Longus	Posterior surface of tibia	Distal phalanges, digits 2, 3, 4, 5	Flexes DIP; plantar flexes and inverts foot	Tibial nerve (L5, S1, 2)
Tibialis Posterior	Tibia; fibula; interosseous membrane	Navicular and adjacent bones	Plantar flexes; inverts foot	Tibial nerve (L4, 5, S1)
Tibialis Anterior	Tibia; interosseous membrane	First cuneiform; first metatarsal	Dorsiflexes, inverts foot	Deep Peroneal nerve (L4, 5, S1)
Extensor Hallucis Longus	Fibula; interosseous membrane	Distal phalanx, hallux	Extends hallux; dorsiflexes, inverts foot	Deep Peroneal nerve (L4, 5, S1)
Extensor Digitorum Longus	Tibia; fibula; interosseous membrane	Second and third phalanges of 2, 3, 4, 5	Extends toes; dorsiflexes and everts foot	Deep Peroneal nerve (L4, 5, S1)
Peroneus Tertius	Fibula; interosseous membrane	Base of 5th metatarsal	Dorsiflexes; everts foot	Deep Peroneal nerve (L5, S1)
Peroneus Longus	Fibula	First metatarsal; first cuneiform	Everts foot; plantar flexes	Superficial Peroneal nerve (L4, 5, S1)
Peroneus Brevis	Fibula	Tuberosity of fifth metatarsal	Everts foot; plantar flexes	Superficial Peroneal nerve (L4, 5, S1)

QUESTIONS FOR REVIEW AND STUDY

1. What is the origin of the small saphenous vein?

The small saphenous vein arises from the lateral aspect of the dorsal venous arch of the foot.

    a. With what nerve or nerves does this vein course up the leg?

a. In the foot, inferior to the lateral malleolus, the sural nerve is closely related to the vein. These are closely approximated in the superficial aspect of the calf. Near the popliteal fossa the vein is closely associated with the medial sural cutaneous nerve and the posterior femoral cutaneous nerve.

    b. Where does this vein terminate?

b. The small saphenous vein ends by draining into the popliteal vein or into the perforating tributaries of the profunda femoris vein.

2. What is the origin of the great saphenous vein?

The great saphenous vein arises from the medial aspect of the dorsal venous arch of the foot.

    a. What nerve accompanies this vein from the knee to the foot?

a. The saphenous nerve, a branch of the femoral nerve. This nerve is sensory to the medial aspect of the calf and medial aspect of foot and great toe (hallux).

3. What sensory nerve supplies the posterior aspect of the calf and the lateral side of the foot? How is this nerve formed?

The sural nerve. Formed by the combination of the medial sural cutaneous nerve and the communicating branch of the lateral sural cutaneous nerve.

4. What is the source and region of distribution of the sensory portion of the superficial peroneal nerve?

Arises from the common peroneal. After supplying the peroneus longus and peroneus brevis the nerve pierces the deep fascia to a superficial position in the distal one-third of the leg. It is sensory to this area of the leg anteriorly, and to the dorsum of the foot.

5. Name the source of motor nerve supply to each of the following muscles:

    a. Medial head, gastrocnemius
    b. Lateral head, gastrocnemius
    c. Popliteus
    d. Soleus
    e. Plantaris
    f. Flexor hallucis longus
    g. Flexor digitorum longus
    h. Tibialis posterior
    I. Peroneus longus
    J. Peroneus brevis
    k. Peroneus tertius
    l. Tibialis anterior
    m. Extensor hallucis longus
    n. Extensor hallucis brevis
    o. Extensor digitorum brevis
    p. Extensor digitorum longus

a. (Posterior) tibial nerve
b. (Posterior) tibial nerve
c. (Posterior) tibial nerve
d. (Posterior) tibial nerve
e. (Posterior) tibial nerve
f. (Posterior) tibial nerve
g. (Posterior) tibial nerve
h. (Posterior) tibial nerve
i. Superficial peroneal
j. Superficial peroneal
k. Deep peroneal
l. Deep peroneal
m. Deep peroneal
n. Deep peroneal
o. Deep peroneal
p. Deep peroneal

6. For each of the following, give its origin and termination.

a. Popliteal artery

a. Origin: Continuation of femoral artery beyond adductor hiatus. Terminates by dividing into anterior and posterior tibial arteries.

b. Popliteal vein

b. Origin: Begins at coalescence of venae comitantes of tibial arteries. Terminates by passing through adductor hiatus, becoming femoral vein.

7. A pedestrian is struck at the lateral aspect of the knee by the bumper of a slowly moving automobile He is observed subsequently by a physician to exhibit "foot-drop. The patient can neither dorsiflex nor evert his foot on the injured side; rather, his foot is held in a plantar flexed position.

a. What nerve is injured?

a. Common peroneal

b. Where is the probable point of injury?

b. Where the nerve passes around the neck of the fibula

c. What muscles are affected?

c. Muscles of the anterior (extensor) and lateral (peroneal) compartments.

d. Why is the foot plantar flexed?

e. Why might the foot also be inverted?

d - e. Because the muscles of the posterior compartment which flex and invert the foot are now unopposed.

8. A child playing in a flower garden falls upon a large cactus, suffering deep penetration of the toxic needles in the anterior aspects of the right forearm and leg. When brought to a clinic several days later, the flexor compartment of the forearm and the anterior compartment of the leg are markedly swollen, discolored and acutely painful. The deep fascia over both compartments might be incised widely in treatment. Why?

Inflammation in the fascial-enclosed compartments, with swelling, causes venous, and then arterial occlusion, with possible resultant death of musculature and nerves. Fascial incision allows relief of the intracompartmental swelling and pressure. Similar procedure is often used in care of bites of venomous creatures.

9. Name the boundaries of the popliteal fossa.

a. Roof

a. Skin, superficial and deep fascia

b. Floor

b. Femur, capsule of knee joint

c. Superolateral boundary

c. Biceps femoris

d. Superomedial boundary

d. Tendons of semitendinosus and semimembranosus

e. Inferolateral boundary

e. Lateral head, gastrocnemius

f. Inferomedial boundary

f. Medial head, gastrocnemius

10. What is found in the popliteal fossa?

Most important: popliteal artery and vein, sciatic nerve (or its two terminal branches). Other structures are short saphenous vein, lymph nodes, fat.

200

11. The femoral artery of a patient has been occluded gradually at the adductor hiatus. Trace at least three routes of collateral flow to the leg.

Example 1. Femoral artery, profunda femoris, last perforating branch, popliteal artery.

Example 2. Femoral artery, lateral femoral circumflex, descending branch, superior lateral genicular artery, popliteal artery.

12. Name the muscles which

    a. Invert the foot:

    a. Flexor digitorum longus; flexor hallucis longus, tibialis posterior; tibialis anterior

    b. Evert the foot:

    b. Extensor digitorum longus; peroneus longus, brevis, tertius

13. What spinal nerve level is primarily responsible for the function of foot inversion?

L4 fibers in the deep peroneal nerve and tibial nerve supply the tibialis anterior and tibialis posterior, respectively.

14. What spinal nerve is the most important in the supply of the extensor hallucis longus?

L5 fibers in the deep peroneal nerve

15. What spinal nerves are principally involved in supply of the dorsiflexors and extensors of the foot?

L4, L5 by deep peroneal nerve

16. What is the primary source of motor fibers to the evertors of the foot?

S1 spinal nerve fibers, carried by the superficial peroneal nerve.

17. The patient is experiencing an inability to evert her foot (making it difficult to walk). She also has anesthesia over most of the dorsum of her foot, except that sensation is normal in the web space between her first and second toes. Other functions and sensation are normal.

    Is her problem due to (?):

    a. L5 spinal nerve lesion
    b. Deep peroneal nerve lesion
    c. Superficial peroneal nerve lesion
    d. Common peroneal nerve lesion

    c. Superficial peroneal nerve lesion. L5 loss would result in weakness of dorsiflexion, not foot eversion. Sensation between first and second toes indicates that L5 and deep peroneal nerves are intact, apparently. Loss of deep peroneal would also result in loss of dorsiflexion and inversion of the foot.

18. The patient complains of pain in the back of her lower limb and under her lateral malleolus. She has demonstrable diminution of her Achilles reflex (when compared with her other lower limb) and weakness in foot eversion. What may be responsible for her problems?

There is a good possibility that she has herniation of the intervertebral disk between L5 and S1, causing stretching or compression of her S1 spinal nerve roots.

LABORATORY IDENTIFICATION CHECK-LIST

The Leg

head of fibula
lateral and medial malleoli
tuberosity of tibia
anterior border of tibia
medial and lateral tibial condyles
ligamentum patellae

great saphenous vein
saphenous nerve
short saphenous vein
sural nerve
   medial sural cutaneous nerve
   communicating branch of lateral sural cutaneous
   nerve

superficial peroneal nerve

boundaries of popliteal fossa
semitendinosus muscle
semimembranosus muscle
medial head of gastrocnemius muscle
lateral head of gastrocnemius muscle

popliteal vein, popliteal artery
fat and lymph nodes of popliteal fossa

superolateral, superomedial genicular arteries
inferolateral, inferomedial genicular arteries
middle genicular artery

relationships of popliteal artery and vein
crural fascia
innervation of medial and lateral heads
   of the gastrocnemius
common peroneal nerve

soleus muscle
plantaris tendon and muscle belly
tendo calcaneus
calcaneus bone

triceps surae muscle
nerve to soleus from tibial division of sciatic

superficial, intermediate and deep muscles
   of posterior compartment of leg

popliteus muscle and its nerve

flexor hallucis longus muscle
flexor digitorum longus muscle

tibialis posterior muscle
anterior tibial artery
posterior tibial artery
peroneal artery

anterior compartment of leg
tibialis anterior muscle
extensor hallucis longus muscle
extensor digitorum longus muscle

peroneus tertius muscle

anterior intermuscular septum

anterior tibial artery in anterior compartment
deep peroneal nerve

lateral compartment of leg
peroneus longus muscle
peroneus brevis muscle
superficial peroneal nerve

DEFINITIONS

Crural, crus [L. *cruris*, the skin, leg]

Fibula [L. *fibula*, a brooch or clasp, especially the needle-like part of a clasp]

Peroneal [Gr. *peronay*, a splinter, something pointed for piercing]
The peroneal muscles attach to the slender, pointed fibula bone.

Plantaris [L. *planta*, the sole of the foot; related to Gr. *platus*, flat]
A term relating to the sole of the foot.

Popliteal [L. *poples*, the ham, the back of the knee]

Soleus [L. *solea*, the sole of the foot]
The name of the muscle comes, apparently, from the shape of this muscle and its resemblance to the similarly named fish.

Tibia [L. *tibia*, a flute or similar wind instrument, a pipe]
Primitive musical instruments were sometimes made from the leg bones of birds or other animals.

CHAPTER 13

THE FOOT

Dorsal Aspect of the Foot

Sensory Nerve Supply. Sensory supply to the dorsum of the foot is provided by:

(1) by the **saphenous nerve** - sensory to the medial side of the foot as far as the ball of the great toe;

(2) by the **sural nerve** - sensory to the lateral side of the foot and fifth toe;

(3) by the **superficial peroneal nerve**, which is sensory to most of the dorsum of the foot and toes;

(4) by the terminal portion of the **deep peroneal nerve**, the sensory distribution of which is confined to the web of skin between the great and second toes.

Numerous communications exist between the saphenous, superficial peroneal and sural nerves in the dorsum of the foot; therefore, loss of any one of these individually may result in little or no sensory deficit.

Veins. The **dorsal venous arch** drains metatarsal veins which, in turn, are formed by the coalescence of digital veins. The small, or lesser saphenous vein arises from the lateral aspect of the venous arch. The great saphenous vein begins in the medial portion of the dorsal venous arch and ascends anterior to the medial malleolus, where it is frequently utilized for venepuncture.

*Study the **osteology of the foot** as seen in Figure 13:1.*

Remove the skin from the foot. The following incisions can be helpful in this procedure:

1) a dorsal longitudinal incision, extending from the ankle to the distal phalanx of the second toe [this is the arbitrary "midline" of the foot];

2) a dorsal transverse incision at the bases of the digits;

(3) a similar transverse incision upon the plantar surface of the foot;

(4) dorsal and plantar longitudinal incisions upon the great toe. The skin can be left upon the lateral three toes unless a more thorough dissection is desired.

*Observe that the skin upon the dorsum of the foot is thin - like that upon the dorsum of the hand. Note also that the thick plantar skin is bound firmly to an underlying thick **planter aponeurosis**, comparable to the palmar aponeurosis of the hand. The skin over weight-bearing areas is particularly thick, such as that over the heel, the lateral side and the "ball" of the foot.*

*Remove all superficial fascia from the dorsum of the foot, preserving the cutaneous nerves and veins. Trace the **saphenous, superficial peroneal** and **sural nerves** into the foot to ascertain their relative positions.*

*Upon the dorsum of the foot, note the **dorsal venous arch**, observing its contributions to the great and small saphenous veins. Following its exposure, you will probably find it necessary to remove most of the smaller tributaries to expose deeper structures.*

Retinacula. The tendons that pass to the dorsum of the foot or into the sole of the foot from the anterior, posterior and lateral compartments are held in place by stout restraining bands, the retinacula. These retinacula are thickened portions of the deep fascia which serve to restrain the tendons and prevent their "bowstringing". Among these are the superior and inferior extensor retinacula, the peroneal retinacula and the flexor retinaculum.

The superior extensor retinaculum is attached to the tibia and fibula just proximal to the malleoli of the ankle. A septum passes deeply from this retinaculum, forming a tunnel medially for the

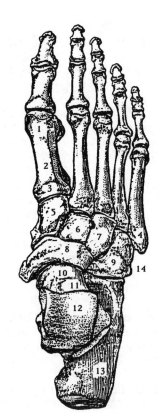

A

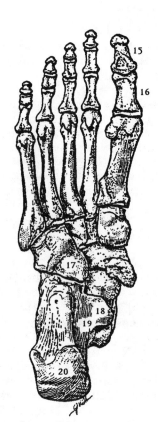

B

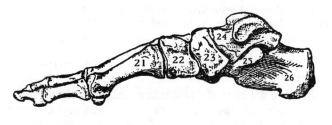

C

D

Figure 13:1 The bones of the foot.

A. Dorsal View
1. Head of first metatarsal
2. Body of first metatarsal
3. Base of first metatarsal
4. Tuberosity of fifth metatarsal
5. First (medial) cuneiform
6. Second (intermediate) cuneiform
7. Third (lateral) cuneiform
8. Navicular
9. Cuboid
10. Head of talus
11. Neck of talus
12. Body {trochlear part} of talus
13. Calcaneus
14. Groove for peroneus longus

B. Plantar Surface
15. Second (distal) phalanx of hallux
16. First (proximal) phalanx of hallux

17. Cuboid
18. Sustentaculum tali of calcaneus
19. Groove for flexor hallucis longus
20. Tuberosity of calcaneus

C. Medial View
21. Base of first metatarsal
22. Medial cuneiform
23. Navicular
24. Head of talus
25. Sustentaculum tali of calcaneus
26. Calcaneus

D. Lateral View
27. Sinus tarsi
28. Trochlea and groove for peroneus longus

passage of the tibialis anterior tendon into the foot, and a lateral tunnel for the entrance of the other extensor tendons.

Extrinsic Muscles of the Dorsum of the Foot. After arising from the anterolateral surface of the tibia and the interosseous membrane, the **tibialis anterior muscle** becomes tendinous at the ankle, passing deep to the extensor retinaculum. Turning medially just beyond the ankle, the tibialis anterior tendon inserts upon the first cuneiform bone and the base of the first metatarsal bone. The tibialis anterior, supplied by the deep peroneal nerve (L4 motor fibers), functions to dorsiflex and invert the foot.

The **extensor hallucis longus** arises from the interosseous membrane and the fibula and inserts upon the great toe. The **extensor digitorum longus** takes origin from the tibia, fibula and the interosseous membrane and gives off tendons to the lateral four toes. The peroneus tertius arises from the fibula, distal to the extensor digitorum longus and inserts upon the base and dorsum of the fifth metatarsal bone. The **peroneus tertius** is considered by some to be derived from the distal portion of the extensor digitorum longus; others consider it a separate, and very important, foot evertor. Like the tibialis anterior, each of these muscles is supplied by the deep peroneal nerve.

In addition to extending the great toe, the extensor hallucis longus dorsiflexes and inverts the foot. The extensor digitorum longus muscle extends the lateral toes, but also - with the peroneus tertius - dorsiflexes and everts the foot.

*Identify the **superior extensor retinaculum**, the "y"-shaped **inferior (cruciate) extensor retinaculum**, **superior** and **inferior peroneal retinacula**, and the **flexor retinaculum** (laciniate ligament).*

*Incise and reflect the retinaculum over the **tibialis anterior** tendon and free up the tendon toward its insertion upon the first cuneiform bone and first metatarsal. Likewise, free up the tendons of the **extensor hallucis longus**, **extensor digitorum longus** and **peroneus tertius** and free them up to their insertions.*

The Extensor Mechanisms of the Digits. As in the hand, the extensor tendons of the toes possess expansions, the "tendinous hoods," which begin at the metatarsophalangeal joints and cover part of the proximal phalanx of each digit. At the distal end of the proximal phalanx of a toe, each tendon divides into three slips - a central, and two lateral bands. The middle tendinous slip inserts upon the middle phalanx of the toe; the lateral bands thereafter unite and insert upon the distal phalanx. The interossei and lumbrical muscles of the foot, like those of the hand, insert partially into the lateral bands, thereby becoming extensors of the interphalangeal joints (because these bands pass dorsal to the transverse axes of these joints).

*Demonstrate the **extensor mechanisms** of the first and second toes. Note that the **extensor hallucis longus** tendon inserts upon the distal (second) phalanx) of the great toe.*

The Peroneus Longus and Peroneus Brevis. The peroneus longus and brevis arise from the fibula. After passing beneath the peroneal retinacula, the peroneus brevis tendon inserts upon the tuberosity of the fifth metatarsal bone; the peroneus longus tendon courses through the sole of the foot, inserting upon the medial cuneiform and first metatarsal bones. Both of these muscles are supplied by the superficial peroneal nerve, with nerve fibers derived almost entirely from the S1 spinal nerve.

*Divide the **superior and inferior peroneal retinacula** over the tendons of the peroneus longus and peroneus brevis. The superior peroneal retinaculum attaches from the lateral malleolus to the calcaneus; the inferior retinaculum attaches across the calcaneus, just below the malleolus. Follow the tendon of the **peroneus brevis** to its insertion upon the tuberosity of the fifth metatarsal bone. Trace the **peroneus longus** tendon to its disappearance into the sole of the foot.*

Study in an Atlas the illustrations of the disposition of the synovial sheaths and tendon sheaths which invest the extrinsic tendons of the dorsum and lateral aspect of the foot.

The Extensor Digitorum Brevis. The extensor digitorum muscle arises from the lateral and distal portions of the calcaneus. The most medial portion of this muscle is commonly named the **extensor hallucis brevis**, inserting upon the great toe. The **extensor digitorum brevis** gives off slender tendons to the second, third and fourth toes. These tendinous slips join the tendons of the extensor digitorum longus for those digits.

*Trace the **extensor hallucis brevis** tendon to its insertion at the base of the proximal phalanx of the great toe. Identify the **extensor digitorum brevis** and trace its tendons to the extensor mechanisms of the other digits.*

The Deep Peroneal Nerve. After distributing branches to the muscles in the anterior compartment, the deep peroneal nerve passes deep to the extensor digitorum brevis - supplying it - and then terminates as a slender ramus which traverses the dorsum of the foot and provides sensory fibers for the region between the first and second toes. The deep peroneal nerve is composed mostly of fibers from L4 and L5.

Identify the **deep peroneal nerve**, in the anterior compartment of the leg. Trace the nerve to the dorsum of the foot, identify its **motor branches** to the **extensor hallucis brevis** and **extensor digitorum brevis** and then clean it to its distribution to the first and second toes.

Arterial Supply. The **anterior tibial artery** enters the anterior compartment of the leg by passing between the tibia and fibula, above the proximal end of the interosseous membrane. It thereafter passes inferiorly through the compartment to the level of the ankle. As this artery crosses the ankle joint it is found to course with the deep peroneal nerve and is renamed the **dorsalis pedis artery.** The pulse of the dorsalis pedis is readily palpable in most individuals. From the dorsalis pedis arise **medial** and **lateral tarsal branches**, an **arcuate branch** (from which arise the lateral metatarsal vessels); a deep plantar branch, and a terminal **first metatarsal branch.**

The peroneal artery lies, for the most part, within the posterior compartment of the leg. However, it gives origin to a number of penetrating branches which assist, especially, in the supply of the lateral compartment.

Distally, the peroneal artery gives off a variably large **perforating branch** which makes its way between the tibia and fibula just proximal to the inferior tibio-fibular articulation of the ankle. This artery can be of considerable importance in collateral supply about the ankle and may even replace the dorsalis pedis. In about fifteen percent of individuals, the dorsalis pedis is essentially absent and the dorsum of the foot is supplied by other collateral vessels, especially by the perforating branch of the peroneal artery.

Trace the **anterior tibial artery** to the level of the malleoli. About two inches proximal to the lateral malleolus of the ankle identify the **perforating branch of the peroneal artery.** On the dorsum of the foot look for, and identify, the branches of the dorsalis pedis artery if they are prominent and readily demonstrable.

Plantar Aspect of the Foot.

The surgeon who operates on the medial aspect of the foot has cause to be aware of the relations of the structures which lie deep to the flexor retinaculum and the order of their appearance from anterior to posterior. A mnemonic device for remembering the relations of these structures as they pass behind the medial malleolus is, "Tom, **D**ick and **a v**ery **n**ervous **H**arry:"

> Tom - **T**ibialis Posterior
> Dick - Flexor **D**igitorum Longus
> And a - Posterior Tibial Artery

Very - Posterior Tibial Venae Comitantes
Nervous - Tibial Nerve
Harry - Flexor Hallucis Longus

Posterior and inferior to the medial malleolus of the ankle, divide and remove the **flexor retinaculum** and the septae derived from it which separate the tendons and the neurovascular elements which pass into the sole. This retinaculum is also called the **laciniate ligament.**

At the level of the medial malleolus, study, and learn the order of appearance of the following structures. From anterior to posterior, clean and identify:

(1) the **tendon of tibialis posterior;**
(2) the **tendon of flexor digitorum longus;**
(3) the **posterior tibial artery** and its **venae comitantes;**
4) the **tibial nerve;**
5) the **flexor hallucis longus.**

Trace the tendon of the tibialis posterior (a plantar flexor and foot invertor) at least as far as its insertion upon the navicular bone . Clean the flexor digitorum longus, the tibial vessels, the tibial nerve and the flexor hallucis longus to their disappearance deep to the **abductor hallucis.**

Nerves and Vessels of the Sole of the Foot. Motor and sensory supply to the sole of the foot is provided by the medial and lateral plantar nerves, branches which arise from the tibial nerve just distal to its passage posterior to the medial malleolus. Vascular supply is provided by the medial and lateral plantar arteries and their venae comitants.

The Plantar Nerves. The medial plantar nerve passes into the sole between the **abductor hallucis** and the **flexor digitorum brevis** and supplies both of these muscles. It also provides rami to the **flexor hallucis brevis** and **first lumbrical** and distributes sensory branches to the plantar surface of the medial three and one-half digits. Thus, the medial plantar nerve innervates only four plantar muscles. The remainder are innervated by the lateral plantar nerve. The medial plantar nerve is comparable to the median nerve of the hand; the lateral plantar nerve is quite similar in distribution to the ulnar nerve.

The **lateral plantar nerve**, after passing deep to the abductor hallucis and flexor digitorum brevis, innervates the **quadratus plantae** and **abductor digiti minimi** and then divides into superficial and deep branches. The **superficial branch** innervates the **flexor digiti minimi brevis** and two interossei and provides sensory supply to the lateral one and one-half digits.

The **deep branch** of the lateral plantar nerve passes into the sole obliquely, deep to the flexor tendons and the **adductor hallucis** supplying this muscle, the three **lumbrical muscles** and **five interossei.**

To recapitulate, the medial plantar nerve is motor to abductor hallucis, flexor digitorum brevis, flexor hallucis brevis and the first lumbrical; it is sensory to three and one-half digits. The lateral plantar nerve innervates all other intrinsic muscles of the sole and is sensory to the lateral one and one-half digits.

Plantar Vessels. The **lateral plantar artery**, the larger terminal branch of the posterior tibial artery, passes with the deep branch of the lateral plantar nerve medially and deep across the sole, forming a deep **plantar arterial arch.** From this arch **metatarsal** and **perforating** branches arise, the metatarsal branches giving origin to plantar digital vessels and the perforating arteries linking the deep arch to the dorsal metatarsal vessels. The terminal portion of the arch is completed by an anastomosis with the plantar branch of the dorsalis pedis artery.

The **medial plantar artery** provides muscular and superficial branches to the medial side of the foot, in addition to several small branches that communicate with the lateral plantar artery.

The Plantar Aponeurosis. This aponeurosis is attached proximally to the calcaneus bone, for the most part. Distally, each of the digital slips divides, passing to either side of the flexor tendons, and contributes to the formation of the fibrous flexor sheath of that digit.

*Subsequent to the removal of skin and superficial fascia from the sole of the foot identify the **plantar aponeurosis** and its fibrous slips to each of the digits. Between the adjacent fibrous slips to the digits from the plantar aponeurosis, identify the **digital vessels** and **nerves.***

*Divide the individual fibrous digital extensions of the plantar aponeurosis, and then reflect the aponeurosis posteriorly to the calcaneus, carefully separating it from the underlying **flexor digitorum brevis muscle.** As this is done, note that...*
*(1) the medial and lateral **plantar fasciae** are considerably thinner than the central aponeurosis;*
*2) longitudinal fibrous **septae** extend deeply from the margins of the aponeurosis;*
(3) a superficial muscle (the flexor digitorum brevis) arises in part from the deep surface of the aponeurosis and must be separated from it with care.

Compartments and Layers of the Sole of the Foot. There are a couple of rather different ways in which the anatomy of the sole of the foot can be presented, studied and learned. By one approach, one considers the deep attachments of the plantar aponeurosis, which effectively separates the tendons, nerves and vessels of the sole into **medial**, **intermediate** and **lateral compartments.** The medial compartment contains, primarily, certain

structures related to the anatomy of the great toe. Similarly, the lateral compartment contains elements related to the fifth toe. All anatomic features in between these two toes are, for the most part, put into the intermediate compartment. This approach to the anatomy is particularly important clinically in compartmental pressure problems or surgical procedures for various purposes.

As one attempts to learn the details of the anatomy of the sole, perhaps the "easiest" approach is to learn its structures - particularly its muscles and tendons - in layers. Four layers are typically described.

First Layer. The first layer of plantar muscles includes the:
  (1) **abductor hallucis** (which inserts on the medial side of the base of the proximal phalanx); the
  (2) **flexor digitorum brevis,** and the
  (3) **abductor digiti minimi** (which inserts on the lateral side of the proximal phalanx).

*Identify and clean the **abductor hallucis**, the most superficial muscle of the medial aspect of the sole. Clean, and trace the tendons of the **flexor digitorum brevis** to the lateral four toes. Upon the lateral side of the sole, identify the **abductor digiti minimi.***

*Divide the abductor hallucis where it covers the entrance of vessels and nerves into the sole. Identify the **medial and lateral plantar nerves** and the **medial** and **lateral plantar arteries**, the terminal divisions of the posterior tibial nerve and artery.*

*Divide the **flexor digitorum brevis** near the calcaneus and reflect it toward the toes. The tendons of this muscle split (for the passage of the tendons of the flexor digitorum longus) before inserting at the bases of the middle phalanges of the lateral four digits.*

*Clean the lateral plantar nerve and vessels in their course deep to the flexor digitorum brevis, to the lateral side of the sole. Look for, and clean, the **superficial** and **deep branches** of the lateral plantar nerve and artery. Identify the **deep plantar arterial arch** and the **deep branch** of the **lateral plantar nerve** and trace them out to their passage beneath the deeper musculature.*

Second Layer of Muscles. The second layer of musculo-tendinous elements includes:
  (1) the **tendon of the flexor hallucis longus,** passing deep, and connected by a tendinous slip, to...
  (2) the **tendon of the flexor digitorum longus;**
  (3) the **quadratus plantae,** or flexor accessorius, a short muscle which arises from the calcaneus and inserts upon the flexor digitorum longus tendon;
  (4) four slender **lumbrical muscles,** which arise from the tendons of the flexor digitorum longus

and insert into the medial aspect of the extensor expansions of the lateral four toes.

The flexor hallucis longus inserts at the base of the last phalanx of the great toe. The flexor digitorum longus inserts by its tendons upon the last phalanx of each of the other toes. The lumbrical muscles insert into the extensor expansions of the medial four digits.

*Identify and mobilize the structures that form the second layer of the muscles of the sole: the **tendons of the flexor hallucis longus, flexor digitorum longus, quadratus plantae** and the **lumbricals**.*

Transect the tendons of the flexor hallucis longus and flexor digitorum longus at the medial aspect of the ankle. To avoid possible confusion in matching the severed tendons, divide one tendon an inch proximal to the other.

*Cut the **tendinous connection between the flexor hallucis longus and flexor digitorum longus**. Sever the attachment of the **quadratus plantae** to the flexor digitorum longus. Reflect the flexor hallucis longus and flexor digitorum longus tendons toward the toes to expose the members of the next layer of musculature.*

Third Layer of Muscles. The third layer of muscles of the sole includes:
    (1) the **flexor hallucis brevis**;
    (2) the **adductor hallucis**;
    (3) the **flexor digiti minimi brevis**.

The **adductor hallucis** possesses an **oblique head** which arises from the bases of the middle metatarsals and a **transverse head** which arises from deep plantar ligaments. The **flexor hallucis brevis** possesses a lateral belly which inserts in common with the adductor hallucis and a medial belly inserting in common with the abductor hallucis.

*Identify the muscles which compose the third layer of the sole: the **flexor hallucis brevis**, the **adductor hallucis** and the **flexor digiti minimi brevis**.*

Fourth Layer of Muscles. The fourth layer of muscle consists of...
    (1) **four dorsal** and
    (2) **three plantar interossei muscles**.
It is more important that the distribution of the interossei be understood than that they should each

be identified. As in the hand, the dorsal interossei abduct, the plantar interossei (cf: palmar interossei) adduct the digits, with respect to the midline. The midline of the foot passes through the second digit. This is different from the hand, in which the midline is designated as passing through the long finger (third digit).

Two dorsal interossei (D1, D2) insert upon the second digit. One dorsal and one plantar interossei (D3, P1) insert upon the third digit; the fourth dorsal and second plantar interossei (D4, P2) insert upon the fourth digit. One plantar interosseous muscle (P3) attaches to the fifth digit.

Identify at least one example of a dorsal and one example of a plantar interosseous muscle.

*Trace the tendon of the peroneus longus medially across the sole to its insertion upon the first cuneiform and first metatarsal bone. Divide the **abductor digiti minimi** to fully expose the peroneus longus tendon, if necessary. Sever the origins and reflect the **flexor digiti minimi brevis** and the oblique head of the **adductor hallucis** to enable you to see the **deep plantar arterial arch** and the branching pattern of the **deep branch of the lateral plantar nerve**.*

QUESTIONS FOR REVIEW AND STUDY

1. What is the innervation of the:

   a. Extensor hallucis brevis
   b. Extensor digitorum brevis
   c. Abductor hallucis
   d. Flexor digitorum brevis
   e. Flexor hallucis brevis
   f. First lumbrical
   g. Quadratus plantae
   h. Abductor digiti minimi
   i. Flexor digiti minimi brevis
   j. Lumbricales 2, 3, 4
   k. Dorsal interossei
   l. Plantar interossei
   m. Adductor hallucis

   a, b: Deep peroneal (or, anterior tibial nerve)

   c - f: Medial plantar nerve, a terminal branch of the posterior tibial nerve

   g - m: Lateral plantar nerve, a terminal branch of the posterior tibial nerve

2. What is the source of sensory supply....

   a. To most of the dorsum of the foot?

   a. Superficial branch of common peroneal

   b. To the lateral side of the dorsum of the foot?

   b. Sural

   c. To the medial side of the dorsum of the foot?

   c. Saphenous nerve

   d. To the plantar aspect of the medial 3 1/2 digits and medial side of the sole?

   d. Medial plantar nerve

   e. To the plantar aspect of the lateral 1 1/2 digits?

   e. Lateral plantar nerve

   f. To the skin between the great and second toe?

   f. Anterior tibial or deep branch, common peroneal

3. The anterior tibial artery is obstructed. Trace two possible routes of collateral arterial supply to the dorsum of the foot.

   (1) Popliteal, posterior tibial, peroneal artery, perforating branch, arteries on dorsum

   (2) Popliteal, posterior tibial, lateral plantar artery, deep plantar arch, perforating branch of first metatarsal artery, dorsalis pedis

4. Name the structures which lie deep to the laciniate ligament, from anterior to posterior.

   Tendon - tibialis posterior
   Tendon - flexor digitorum longus
   Posterior tibial artery
   Tibial nerve
   Tendon - flexor hallucis longus

5. To what non-bony structures does the flexor digitorum longus attach?

   Tendon of flexor hallucis longus; quadratus plantae; lumbricales

6. What major neurovascular structures can be found deep to the adductor hallucis?

   The deep branch of the lateral plantar nerve and the plantar arterial arch.

7. What muscle inserts in common with the abductor hallucis?

   The medial belly of flexor hallucis brevis.

LABORATORY IDENTIFICATION CHECK-LIST

The Foot

OSTEOLOGY OF THE FOOT:

proximal, middle and distal phalanges
metatarsal bones
  base, body, head
  tuberosity of fifth metatarsal
first, second and third cuneiform bones

cuboid bone
  groove for peroneus longus

navicular bone

talus
  body
    trochlear portion for tibial articulation
    sulcus tali for tarsal sinus and interosseous
      ligament
    groove for flexor hallucis longus tendon
    neck
    head
      facet for navicular articulation

calcaneus
  tuberosity for tendo calcaneus
  articular facets
  peroneal trochlea and groove for peroneus longus
  sustentaculum tali and groove for flexor hallucis
    longus
  calcaneal sulcus for tarsal sinus and interosseous
    ligament

DISSECTION FEATURES:

dorsal venous arch of foot
lesser saphenous vein
great saphenous vein

saphenous nerve in foot
superficial peroneal nerve in foot
sural nerve in foot

superior extensor retinaculum
inferior extensor retinaculum
superior and inferior peroneal retinacula
flexor retinaculum

tendon of tibialis anterior
tendons of extensor digitorum longus and extensor
  expansions
tendon of extensor hallucis longus and extensor
  expansion

peroneus tertius tendon

insertion of peroneus brevis muscle

extensor hallucis brevis muscle and tendon
extensor digitorum brevis muscle and tendons
deep peroneal nerve on dorsum of foot and at
  termination
motor branches of deep peroneal nerve on foot

dorsalis pedis artery
perforating branch of peroneal artery

order of structures on medial side of ankle: review
abductor hallucis muscle

plantar aponeurosis

digital vessels and nerves

flexor digitorum brevis muscle
abductor digiti minimi muscle
medial and lateral plantar artery and nerves

tendon of flexor hallucis longus in foot
tendons of flexor digitorum longus in foot
quadratus plantae muscle
lumbrical muscles (four)

flexor hallucis brevis muscle
flexor digiti minimi brevis muscle
oblique and transverse heads of adductor hallucis
  muscle

dorsal interossei muscles (4)
plantar interossei muscles (3)

tendon of peroneus longus at insertion
deep branch of lateral plantar nerve
plantar arterial arch

DEFINITIONS

Cuneiform [L. cuneus, wedge + *forma,* form]
Shaped like a wedge.

Metatarsus [Gr., *meta-* between + *tarsos,* tarsus]
The part of the foot between the tarsus and the toes, its skeleton being five long bones (the metatarsals) extending from the tarsus to the phalanges.

Navicular [L., *navicula,* boat]
Boat-shaped, as the navicular bone.

Phalanx (pl. phalanges) [Gr., *phalanx,* "a line or array of soldiers]
A general term for any bone of a finger or toe.

Retinaculum (pl. retinacula) [L., retinaculum -" a rope cable"]
A general term for a structure which retains an organ or tissue in place.

Sustentaculum tali [L., *sustentare,* to hold up or support + *talus,* heel or ankle]
A process of the calcaneus which supports the talus.

Talus (pl. tali) [L. "ankle"]
The most proximal of the tarsal bones and the one which articulates with the tibia and fibula to form the ankle joint.

CHAPTER 14

THE ARTICULATIONS OF THE LOWER MEMBER

In this dissection, special attention should be given to the morphology of the hip joint and knee joint. In addition, two primary ligaments associated with the stability of the foot should be demonstrated, the deltoid and "spring" ligaments. To obtain the most lasting and pragmatic benefits from this exercise, take some time to study the bony and ligamentous features of the joints as depicted in an Atlas before attempting the dissection

The Hip Joint

The hip joint, a ball and socket joint, is the strongest joint in the body. Strength is imparted to it by (1) overlying muscles; (2) the strong stabilizing ligaments; (3) intracapsular negative pressure. If the muscles which surround the hip joint are removed in an unembalmed body, the joint resists dislocation. If a hollow cannula is introduced into the capsule, however, allowing outside air to enter the joint, it becomes dislocated quite readily. The hip joint is weakest inferiorly, like the shoulder.

In order to increase the mobility of the extremity for subsequent procedures, the hip joint will be the first joint to be dissected. Although some muscles will require removal to expose the hip (and other) joints, the vessels and nerves should be left intact as much as possible, the better to understand their anatomic relations to the joints and the possibilities of neurovascular complications in dislocations and fractures.

The proximity of the femoral vessels and nerve to the hip joint is of considerable significance in surgical procedures of the hip joint, for they are separated from the joint solely by the iliopsoas. A nail driven upward through the neck of the femur in orthopedic procedures can easily result in neural or vascular damage if it is misdirected and driven too far anteriorly.

In about ten per cent of individuals the bursa which lies beneath the iliopsoas muscle communicates with the synovial cavity of the hip joint.

To expose the ligaments of the anterior aspect of the capsule of the hip joint it will first be necessary to remove or reflect aside the inguinal ligament and several muscles. The first of these is the **iliopsoas**. This muscle, a combination of the iliacus and psoas major arises from the iliac fossa and the lumbar vertebrae. The thick, muscular tendon passes inferiorly and laterally around the articular capsule of the joint to insert upon the lesser trochanter.

Second, the **sartorius** arises from the anterior superior iliac spine and crosses the length of the thigh obliquely, from anterior to medial before inserting upon the tibia. Third, the **rectus femoris** has two rather distinct sites of origin from the hip bone. The more obvious origin is the anterior inferior iliac spine. Posteriorly, a second tendon arises just above the acetabulum and travels forward to join the tendon arising from the anterior inferior iliac spine. The combined rectus tendon joins the other tendons of the quadriceps femoris distally in the anterior compartment of the thigh. Finally, the **tensor fasciae latae** muscle arises from the lateral and anterior portion of the iliac crest. Its tendinous fibers join those of the gluteus maximus which insert by means of the iliotibial tract on the lateral aspect of the tibia, proximally.

Dissection

*Remove the **inguinal ligament** on the right side of the cadaver. Review the position and significance of the femoral vessels and nerve and the femoral sheath. With the scalpel, sever the **right psoas major** and **iliacus** muscles at the level of the inguinal ligament. Attempt to identify the **iliopsoas bursa**. Turn the combined iliopsoas tendon distally, toward its insertion upon the lesser trochanter. Leave the femoral vessels, femoral nerve and medial femoral circumflex artery intact in this procedure.*

*Transect the tendon of origin of the **sartorius** at its attachment to the anterior superior iliac spine and then reflect the muscle inferiorly. Similarly, but more carefully, cut the tendon of the **rectus femoris** away from the anterior inferior iliac spine while looking for its more inferior tendon of origin, which arises from*

214

the brim of the acetabulum, the **reflected head of the rectus femoris**. Secure, and preserve the tendon of the reflected head. Its posterior extent will be more easily seen when the body has been turned to the prone position.

Divide the **tensor fasciae latae muscle** at its bony origin from the anterior part of the iliac crest. After retracting the iliopsoas tendon downward, inspect the anterior portion of the capsule of the hip joint. [It may be necessary to carefully scrape away some adipose and other connective tissue before you will be able to see the dense fibrous capsule.]

You should be able to see the head of the femur, covered only by an extremely thin, translucent portion of the capsule, in the vicinity of the psoas bursa. Reflect the pectineus muscle inferiorly from its origin to expose the medial aspect of the joint capsule more clearly.

Ligaments of the Hip. Three ligaments are particularly important in thickening the articular capsule and providing strength to the articulation. These include the **iliofemoral**, **pubofemoral** and **ischiofemoral ligaments.** The most important of these is the iliofemoral ligament, one of the strongest ligaments of the body. It helps to prevent hyperextension of the hip joint. The ischiofemoral ligament helps prevent excessive medial rotation of the femur.

Anteriorly, two thickened ligamentous portions of the fibrous capsule will now be identified:

(1) the inverted "Y" or "V" -shaped **iliofemoral ligament,** (the so-called Ligament of Bigelow) extending from the anterior inferior iliac spine toward the greater trochanter and intertrochanteric line;

(2) the **pubofemoral ligament,** extending from the medial portion of the superior pubic ramus to the femur above the iliopsoas insertion.

Place the cadaver in the prone (face down) position. Remove the gluteus medius and gluteus minimus by dividing their tendinous insertions upon the greater trochanter. From this position, beginning near the anterior inferior iliac spine it will be a simple matter to identify the **reflected tendon** of origin of the rectus femoris, which contributes some fibers to the joint capsule near the brim of the acetabulum.

Divide the tendons of the piriformis, obturator internus, quadratus femoris and obturator externus at their insertions.

Posteriorly, identify the **ischiofemoral ligament** - the posterior ligament strengthening the fibrous joint capsule. Scrape away any connective tissue or muscular fibers which may conceal the posterior inferior portion of the joint capsule near the junction of the femoral neck and the greater trochanter.

Confirm the fact that the joint capsule is not attached directly to bone in this region. Make an incision in the capsule, parallel with the orientation of the femoral neck; open the capsule and look within for vessels which enter the joint capsule in this region.

With the overlying muscles removed and the capsule yet intact, except for the above incision, move the femur through flexion, extension, abduction, adduction, medial and lateral rotation and circumduction of the hip joint.

The Acetabulum. The acetabulum, the socket of the hip joint, consists of...

(1) an articular cavity with a hyaline cartilage covered **lunate surface**, the bony rim of which is thickened by overlying cartilage to form the **acetabular labrum**. The bony rim has a deep **acetabular notch** in it, inferiorly. The part of the labrum which passes across the notch, the **transverse acetabular ligament**, converts the notch into an **acetabular foramen**.

(2) a non-articular, rough-surfaced **acetabular fossa**, occupied by fat, blood vessels and the **ligament of the head of the femur**.

The **ligament of the femoral head** does little to stabilize the head of the femur; rather, it conveys important blood vessels to the head of the femur in early life; that is, until about the age of eight years. Thereafter, the artery becomes reduced in size and relatively insignificant in vascular supply to the bone. The ligamentum teres femoris is attached inferiorly to the transverse ligament, which bridges the acetabular notch.

Blood Supply of the Hip Joint. The arterial supply for the head and neck of the femur is derived primarily from rather small branches of the femoral circumflex and the gluteal arteries. These small vessels enter these parts of the bone by passing deep to the arching, loose posterior portion of the capsule of the hip joint. Thereafter, they enter the neck by numerous nutrient foramina and pass toward the head of the femur. In a fracture of the femoral neck, it is these vessels which may be torn, depriving the neck and head of their blood supply.

The **artery to the head of the femur** (the "foveolar artery"), usually a branch of the **obturator artery**, passes with the ligamentum teres to attain the femoral head. Because collateral vessels from the neck of the femur, which are derived from the circumflex and gluteal vessels, do not usually have adequate anastomoses with the vessels that supply the femoral head directly, interruption of the supply to the head can result in its necrosis (as happens often in fractures of the neck of the femur).

Extend the capsular incision to the edge of the acetabulum, and then broadly incise the superior and posterior aspects of the fibrous capsule adjacent to the bony rim of the acetabulum. Rotate the femur medially to bring the head of the femur fully into view.

Identify the thick, fibrocartilaginous **acetabular labrum**, which deepens the articular cavity and observe the cartilage covered **lunate (articular) surface** of the acetabulum. Note the cluster of fat and blood vessels deeply within the acetabulum in the **non-articular acetabular fossa**.

Attaching to a depressed area on the head of the femur, the **fovea capitis**, identify the **ligamentum teres**. Subsequently, identify the **transverse acetabular ligament** at the **acetabular foramen**.

Deep to the transverse ligament, in the acetabular foramen, identify the **artery to the head of the femur**.

The Knee Joint

The knee joint is the largest joint in the body. The synovial cavity of this joint is likewise the largest in the body. The knee is a hinge-type, diarthrodial joint, but it also possesses some rotatory function as well. Passage from the flexed position of the joint into extension involves a forward gliding, rolling and medial rotation of the femur upon the tibia. The cruciate ligaments, the shapes of the approximating surfaces of the tibia and femur, and the mobility of the menisci are all of significance in the "locking mechanism" of the knee joint in extension. In addition, the cruciate ligaments aid in preventing forward or backward displacement of the femur and tibia upon one another.

Bursae of the Knee. Approximately twelve bursae are found in relation to the knee. Two of these are **subcutaneous** in position. The subcutaneous **prepatellar bursa** is frequently involved in a bursitis called "housemaid's knee". A subcutaneous **infrapatellar bursa** is likewise occasionally involved in "parson's knee" bursitis. Pain in such inflammations can be quite intense.

Ligaments of the Knee. The deep fascia upon the anterior, medial and lateral aspects of the knee is strengthened by diverging fibers of the tendons that insert about this joint, principally the quadriceps. This thickened, very strong fascia is called, upon the medial and lateral aspects of the knee, respectively, the **medial** and **lateral retinacula** of the knee.

The ligaments of the knee joint which will be exposed in this dissection include the **medial collateral ligament**, the **lateral collateral ligament**, the **anterior and posterior cruciate ligaments** and several other bands which appear as thickenings of the articular capsule. In addition, we shall also see the medial and lateral meniscal cartilages of the knee joint.

The **tibial collateral ligament** is a somewhat deltoid-shaped band which joins the medial and lateral condyles of the femur and tibia. The tibial collateral ligament is attached by its deeper layer of fibers to the medial semilunar cartilage (medial meniscus) of the knee joint. The cartilage itself is attached to the edge of the tibial plateau by the so-called coronary ligament. For this reason, when the lateral aspect of the weight-bearing knee is struck with considerable force (as in "clipping" in football), the tibial or medial collateral ligament may be damaged and the medial internal cartilage of the knee joint may be torn at the same time.

Because the medial retinaculum is partially continuous with the **tibial collateral ligament**, reference should be made frequently to an Atlas for the position and extent of the tibial collateral ligament, to avoid its destruction when dissecting away the retinaculum.

The **fibular collateral ligament** is a very stout, cord-like band that passes from the lateral femoral epicondyle to the head of the fibula. This ligament lies deep to the iliotibial tract and external to the capsule of the knee joint. Its fibers are intimately related to the tendon of the biceps femoris at its fibular insertion.

The meniscal, or semilunar, cartilages of the knee joint are fibrocartilaginous pads which serve to deepen the articular surfaces of the tibia to receive the condyles of the femur. The **medial meniscus** is semicircular in form and, as noted above, is joined peripherally to the medial collateral ligament.

The **lateral meniscus** is more circular in form than the medial meniscus. It is more mobile than the medial meniscus, moving with the lateral femoral condyle in knee flexion and extension. It has attachments to the popliteus muscle and to the posterior cruciate ligament which may be of some functional importance in joint movement.

The anterior cruciate ligament and posterior cruciate ligament join the tibia and femur together within the knee joint. Although they are within the joint, they are covered with synovial membrane and are thereby separated from the intraarticular space. The **anterior cruciate ligament** passes upward and laterally from the anterior medial aspect of the tibial plateau to reach the posterior part of the medial surface of the lateral femoral condyle.

The **posterior cruciate ligament** attaches to a depression behind the intraarticular surface of the tibia inferiorly and to the lateral surface of the medial femoral condyle. This ligament is joined to the lateral meniscus of the joint by means of the **meniscofemoral ligament**.

216

Dissection.

Medially, trace the tendons of the sartorius, gracilis and semitendinosus to their common insertion, inferior and medial to the tuberosity of the tibia. The morphology of this tendinous insertion has led to the name **pes anserinus** *(goose foot).*

Identify and define the tendons of the quadriceps femoris and semimembranosus. Excise the medial retinaculum to expose the **tibial collateral ligament**. *This extrinsic ligament is a broad band closely applied to the capsule of the joint and attaches from the medial epicondyle of the femur to the medial tibial condyle.*

Note that the shorter, more posterior, fibers of the tibial collateral ligament attach to the tibia, deep to, and proximal to, the semimembranosus insertion. As noted before, these fibers are important in binding the medial meniscus to the tibia.

Make an incision lateral and medial to the quadriceps tendon, patella and ligamentum patella and then transect the ligamentum patella. Reflect the patella and its ligaments superiorly to expose the anterior internal features of the knee joint.

As the quadriceps tendon is reflected, identify the **suprapatellar** *and* **deep infrapatellar bursae** *deep to the quadriceps tendon and ligamentum patella. Identify the* **infrapatellar fat pad***; expose it, and remove sufficient synovial tissue to demonstrate the* **anterior cruciate ligament** *and the* **menisci**. *The anterior cruciate ligament assists in prevention of hyperextension of the knee and posterior gliding of the femur on the fixed tibia.*

Laterally, identify the tendon of the biceps femoris. Trace the tendon to the head of the fibula and then divide it at its bony attachment. With the biceps tendon removed, identify the major lateral extrinsic ligament of the knee, the strong, cordlike **fibular collateral ligament** *which passes between the lateral femoral condyle and the head of the fibula.*

Posterior to the knee, the fibrous capsule is rather thin. However, observe the contributions to the fibrous capsule in this area afforded by expansions from the semimembranosus tendon and ligamentous tissues (the **arcuate ligament**) *associated with the* **popliteus muscle**.

Cut the tendon of the **semimembranosus** *just proximal to its tibial insertion, leaving the very distal end of the tendon intact, to better appreciate the contribution of its fibers to the capsule of the knee joint. Remove connective tissues and other muscles which obscure the posterior aspect of the knee joint, but preserve the major vessels and nerves of the popliteal fossa.*

The **popliteus muscle** passes through the capsule of the knee joint. In its course, the popliteus attaches to the lateral meniscus. The significance of this fact is explained by some orthopedists as follows. During the process of knee extension, the lateral condyle of the femur at first rolls, and then slides forward, dragging the lateral meniscus with it until the medial rotation of the femur upon the tibial condyle is halted and the joint locks in position. When flexion of the knee is initiated, contraction of the popliteus begins the reversal of direction of the femur and, at the same time, pulls the lateral meniscus posteriorly - so that it is not crushed beneath the encroaching lateral femoral condyle.

Incise the posterior aspect of the fibrous capsule transversely and dissect away enough of the fibrous tissue to expose the intrinsic ligaments of the knee; the **lateral** *and* **medial menisci** *(semilunar cartilages), the* **posterior cruciate ligament** *and the* **meniscofemoral ligament**. *The meniscofemoral ligament is a fibrous cord that arises from the lateral meniscus and blends with the posterior cruciate ligament.*

Note that the posterior cruciate ligament becomes taut when the knee is flexed. This ligament prevents the femur from sliding too far forward upon the articular surface of the tibia when the tibia is fixed. It will be more readily seen, when the anterior aspect of the knee joint is open, that the anterior cruciate ligament becomes taut when the knee is in full extension - thus explaining why it is torn when the extended knee is hit forcibly from a posterolateral direction.

Nerve Supply. The nerve supply about the knee is contributed by the femoral nerve (by a large infrapatellar branch of the saphenous nerve), the lateral femoral cutaneous nerve, and additional rami to the joint from the sciatic and obturator nerves. Remember this general principle: "The nerve which supplies a joint supplies also the muscles which move the joint and the skin covering the articular insertion of these muscles" (**Hilton's law**).

Tibiofibular Articulations

The fibula is connected throughout its length to the tibia by two joints and by the interosseous membrane. These joints are constructed so as to maintain the relationship of the tibia to the fibula and also to provide stability to the knee and ankle joints.

1. **The proximal tibiofibular** articulation is a gliding type of synovial joint where movement occurs between both the tibia and fibula. The articular capsule of this joint is very strong, especially anteriorly and posteriorly, where it is thickened by the anterior and posterior superior tibiofibular ligaments.

217

2. The **middle tibiofibular** articulation is represented by an **interosseous membrane** which attaches along the lengths of the shafts of the tibia and fibula. A gap in the proximal part of the membrane allows for passage of the anterior tibial vessels and a gap in the distal end transmits the perforating branch of the peroneal artery.

3. The **distal tibiofibular joint** is classified as a **fibrous (syndesmosis)** type of articulation. The strength of the capsule and ligaments permit a slight gliding of the fibula on the tibia in a longitudinal direction.

Identify the proximal and distal tibiofibular ligaments and the interosseous membrane, removing or reflecting connective tissues and muscles as necessary. Remember to attempt to preserve the major nerves and vessels.

Ankle Joint and Joints of the Foot

The joints of the ankle and foot are subject to many postural and traumatic problems and to various disease processes; thus they actually merit more study than will be given here. **Inversion sprains** (tearing of the calcaneofibular and anterior talofibular ligaments) and, less commonly, **eversion sprains** (damage to deltoid ligament), for instance, are among the most ordinary of injuries. It is to be hoped that this initial study, although brief, will stimulate further investigation at a later time on the part of the interested student.

The **ankle joint** is a relatively simple, hinge-type (**ginglymus**) joint formed by the tibia and fibula proximally, and the **talus** bone distally. [**Inversion and eversion of the foot take place through intertarsal joints, not the ankle** (talocrural) **joint.**]

Three ligaments act together to form the lateral ligamentous unit of the ankle. These include the **anterior talofibular ligament**, the **calcaneofibular ligament** and the **posterior talofibular ligament**. Of these three parts, the posterior talofibular ligament is the strongest. The anterior talofibular ligament is probably the most important clinically in that, if it is torn, considerable lateral instability results. The anterior talofibular ligament and the calcaneofibular ligament are the most commonly involved ligaments in sprains.

The **interosseous talocalcaneal ligament** is the chief bond of union between the talus and calcaneus bones. It is rather centrally located, lying almost hidden between the two bones in the **tarsal sinus**.

*Identify the **anterior talofibular ligament**, the **calcaneofibular ligament**, and the **posterior talofibular ligament**. You will first need to remove any remnants of the extensor retinacula and the peroneal retinacula. Take care in removing the* retinacula which bind the tendons of the peroneus longus and brevis to the fibula and calcaneus, because the calcaneofibular ligament lies just deep to the superior peroneal retinaculum. Reflect the tendinous origin of the extensor digitorum brevis to assist you in finding the **interosseous talocalcaneal ligament** *laterally in the foot.*

The **deltoid ligament** (medial collateral ligament) is the principal ligament upon the medial side of the ankle region. It is composed of **anterior tibiotalar, tibionavicular, tibiocalcaneal** and **posterior tibiotalar** components, each of which is a strong ligament in itself and contributes to the overall integrity of the deltoid ligament.

To expose the deltoid ligament, divide the tendons of the tibialis anterior and tibialis posterior an inch or so proximal to their insertions and remove the synovium and connective tissue sheaths which are usually quite adherent to the underlying fibers of the ligament.

A number of important ligaments on the plantar surface of the foot not only help to maintain the integrity of the bony articulations but also provide strong support for the arches of the foot. These include the **plantar calcaneonavicular ligament**, the **long plantar ligament** and the **short plantar ligaments**.

The **plantar calcaneonavicular ligament** extends from the sustentaculum tali to the navicular bone and is an important structure in the maintenance of the **longitudinal arch** of the foot. When the talus bone receives the weight of the body, transmitted through the ankle, the head of the talus is supported principally by this "spring" ligament, between the calcaneus and navicular bones.

The **long plantar ligament** crosses the tendon of the peroneus longus as the peroneal tendon is making its way to insertion medially on the base of the first metatarsal. This ligament passes from the calcaneus to attach to the cuboid and the bases of the lateral three metatarsals. The **short plantar ligament** is easily confused with the spring ligament; it diverges medially from the long plantar ligament and attaches to the cuboid bone - not the navicular bone.

*Identify the **plantar calcaneonavicular** or "spring" ligament. It may be found lateral, and deep to, the proximal portion of the insertion of the tibialis posterior.*

*The long and short plantar ligaments are easily found after the deeper muscles of the sole of the foot and underlying connective tissue are removed. Lateral to the calcaneonavicular ligament, identify the **long plantar** and **short plantar ligaments**.*

The lever function performed by the feet in propelling, and bearing the weight of the body is assisted by resilient **longitudinal** and **transverse arches.** The longitudinal arch (sometimes described as separate medial and lateral longitudinal arches) is a long curve passing through the heel (calcaneus), the head of the talus ("keystone"), the navicular bone, the three cuneiforms and the heads of the medial three metatarsal bones. The longitudinal arch is supported by:

(1) the spring ligament;
(2) the plantar aponeurosis;
(3) the long plantar ligament;
(4) the tendons of the tibialis posterior and
  peroneus longus.

The **transverse arch of the foot** completes the "domed" appearance of the middle of the sole, presenting a side-to-side curve from the heads of the metatarsals distally, to the navicular and cuboid bones, proximally. The transverse arch is maintained by:

(1) the adductor hallucis and
(2) by plantar intertarsal and tarsometatarsal ligaments.

Failure or compromise of this arch produces pain by pressure upon digital nerves and vessels.

QUESTIONS FOR REVIEW AND STUDY

1. What is the insertion of the common tendon of the iliopsoas (iliacus, plus psoas major)?

Lesser trochanter

What is the function of the iliopsoas?

Flexion of the hip

2. What are the origin, insertion and innervation of the sartorius?

O: Anterior superior iliac spine
I: Medial side of proximal end of tibia
N: Femoral nerve

3. What are the origin, insertion and innervation of the rectus femoris?

O: Anterior inferior iliac spine and reflected origin from area adjacent to the brim of the acetabulum.
I: Inserts with other quadriceps femoris muscles through patella to tibial tuberosity.
N: Femoral nerve. Extends the knee joint.

4. What separates the femoral nerve and vessels from the hip joint?

Principally, muscle and tendon of the iliopsoas.

5. What are the insertion, function and innervation of the pectineus?

I: Pectineal line
F: Hip flexion and adduction
N: Femoral or accessory obturator and adduction

6. What are the three major ligaments of the hip joint?

Pubofemoral, iliofemoral, ischiofemoral.

7. What is the function of the "Y-shaped ligament (of Bigelow)"?

Prevents hyperextension of the femur.

8. What is the function of the ischiofemoral ligament?

Helps prevent excessive medial rotation of the femur.

9. Name the two parts of the acetabular fossa.

The lunate (articular) surface and the nonarticular, acetabular fossa.

10. What is the name of the fibrocartilaginous rim of the acetabulum?

Acetabular labrum

11. What is the name of the depressed area on the femoral head? What attaches at this point?

Fovea capitis. Ligamentum teres (ligament of the head of the femur)

12. What is the function of the ligamentum teres capitis femoris?

Conveys blood vessels for supply of the head of the femur (primarily in childhood)

13. The _____ ligament bridges the acetabular notch converting it into the_____.

Acetabular ligament. Acetabular foramen. Contains the vessels to the head of the femur, usually the obturator artery.

14. What features provide strength and stability to the hip joint?

(1) Overlying muscles; (2) the ligaments of the capsule; (3) intracapsular negative pressure.

15. What aspect of the hip joint is the weakest?

Like the shoulder joint, its inferior aspect.

16. What is the composition of the medial and lateral retinacula of the knee?

Deep fascia, combined with tendinous fibers from muscles associated with the knee, particularly the quadriceps, biceps and iliotibial tract.

17. What is the origin, insertion and innervation of the long head of the biceps femoris?

O: Ischial tuberosity
I: Head of the fibula
N: Tibial division of the sciatic nerve.

18. What bony points are connected by the fibular collateral ligament?

Lateral femoral condyle and head of the fibula.

19. Name the three muscles which insert just medial to the tibial tuberosity. Name another characteristic common to these muscles. Name a feature upon which they differ from one another.

By the pes anserinus: the sartorius, gracilis and semitendinosus. Each of these muscles crosses two joints. Each is supplied by a different nerve.

20. What is a sesamoid bone?

Sesamoid bones are bones which develop within tendons, where these tendons are subject to both pressure and tensile stress. These are consistent enough in number to be considered part of the bony skeleton, and there are usually more in the fetus than in the adult. Sesamoid bones are particularly numerous in the palmar aspect of the hand and in the plantar portion of the foot.

21. What is the largest sesamoid bone?

The patella

22. What is the clinical importance of sesamoid bones?

On X-ray, a sesamoid bone may be mistakenly believed to be a displaced portion of a fractured bone, by the unsuspecting. Second, sesamoid bones have no periosteum. Therefore, in fractures of the patella, for example, the bony union of the healing fragments is mostly fibrous, and can take place only at the fractured surfaces. Careful reapproximation of the parts of a broken patella must be done for healing to take place.

23. What is the innervation of the knee joint?

"Hilton's law" states, in effect, that the nerves innervating the muscles which move a joint also innervate the joint. The knee joint is innervated by nerve rami from the obturator, femoral and sciatic nerves.

24. What is the innervation of the hip joint?

The hip joint is innervated from the same nerves as the knee joint. The clinical importance of this rests in the fact that pain can be "referred" from the hip joint to the knee joint, or vice versa. A patient complaining of a painful knee joint should be carefully examined also for possible disease of the hip joint.

25. What are the three "C's" in examinations of the knee joint?

Examination of the Collateral ligaments, the Cruciate ligaments and of the Cartilages (menisci).

26. What is the "unhappy triad" in injury of the knee joint?

Injury to the anterior cruciate ligament; tibial collateral ligament, and the medial meniscus. The anterior cruciate ligament tightens in extension of the knee. Anterior displacement of the tibia, with respect to its articulation with the femur, can damage this ligament. The tibial (medial) collateral ligament is attached to the medial meniscus; thus, the frequent simultaneous injury to both these ligaments.

27. What is the function of the posterior cruciate ligament?

It tightens in flexion of the knee. It can be damaged by posterior displacement of the tibia upon the femur.

28. What is the significance of the prepatellar bursa and infrapatellar bursa?

Both bursae may become inflamed and painful; the prepatellar bursitis (housemaid's knee) and infrapatellar bursitis (parson's knee) occur from frequent pressure against a hard surface.

29. What bones take part in the formation of the ankle joint?

The tibia and fibula proximally, the talus (astragalus) distally.

30. What joints are involved in eversion and inversion of the foot?

Intertarsal joints, particularly those between the talus, navicular and calcaneus.

31. Name the parts of the deltoid ligament.

Anterior talotibial; tibionavicular; calcaneotibial; posterior talotibial ligaments.

32. What's the most important supportive ligament of the foot?

Probably the plantar calcaneonavicular ("spring") ligament.

33. What is the function of the deltoid ligament?

One important function is the prevention of overeversion of the ankle. The ligament is so strong that excessive eversion may cause the medial malleolus to be pulled off, rather than tearing the deltoid ligament.

34. What bones contribute to the medial longitudinal arch of the foot?

Calcaneus, talus, navicular, three cuneiforms and three medial metatarsals.

35. What composes the lateral bony arch of the foot?

Calcaneus, cuboid, two lateral metatarsals.

36. What forms the transverse arch of the foot?

The wedge-like shapes of middle and lateral cuneiforms and the 2nd, 3rd, and 4th metatarsals.

37. What are the principal factors in support of the arches of the foot?

Primarily the bony architecture and plantar soft tissues. The plantar ligaments and the plantar aponeurosis give passive, but powerful support. Some muscles help to distribute the weight (especially peroneus longus, tibialis anterior and posterior, flexor digitorum longus and flexor hallucis longus).

38. What is the blood supply of the head of the femur?

In the young, of less than about eight years, the artery to the head - which usually arises from the obturator artery. In the adult this artery is of less importance, the blood supply arising from radicular branches of the medial and lateral femoral circumflex.

39. What is the clinical significance of the radicular branches of the medial and lateral femoral circumflex arteries?

These vessels reach the femoral head by passing into the fibrous articular capsule at the distal end of the neck. In fracture of the anatomic neck of the femur these vessels may be lost, with resulting avascular necrosis of the femoral head.

40. How does the obturator artery supply the head of the femur in the young?

An obturator branch passes with the ligamentum teres to the fovea capitis.

41. What is the blood supply of the shaft of the femur (the nutrient artery)?

Usually by the second perforating branch of the profunda femoris (sometimes the 1st or 3rd).

222

42. What is the blood supply of the tibia?

A branch of the posterior tibial artery, the largest such nutrient artery in the body.

43. Name the artery that appears....

a. Between the piriformis and gluteus medius

a. Superior gluteal

b. Between the piriformis and obturator internus.

b. Inferior gluteal

c. Between the obturator internus and quadratus.

c. The ascending branch of the medial femoral circumflex; it provides rami to the greater trochanter and neck of the femur and anastomoses with the ascending branch of the lateral femoral circumflex artery.

d. Between the quadratus femoris and adductor magnus

d. The descending branch of the medial femoral circumflex artery; it gives off branches to the hamstrings, the sciatic nerve and the anastomosis with the first perforating artery and inferior gluteal artery.

e. Through the adductor magnus

e. Perforating branches of profunda femoris

f. Through the adductor hiatus

f. The popliteal artery

g. Between the tibia and fibula proximally, by passing over the upper end of the interosseous membrane

g. Anterior tibial

h. Between the tibia and fibula distally

h. Perforating branch of the peroneal artery.

44. Does the anterior tibial artery get to the anterior muscular compartment by passing around the neck of the fibula (with the common peroneal nerve)?

No. The anterior tibial artery enters the anterior compartment by passing between the tibia and fibula proximally. This relationship is similar to that of the posterior interosseous artery and deep radial nerve in the forearm.

45. What is the importance of the perforating branch of the peroneal artery?

It may replace the dorsalis pedis in the supply of the dorsum of the foot. The dorsalis pedis pulse then appears to be absent due to occlusive disease.

LABORATORY IDENTIFICATION CHECK-LIST

Articulations of the Lower Member

inguinal ligament
iliofemoral ligament
pubofemoral ligament
ischiofemoral ligament

reflected tendon of the rectus femoris muscle

labrum
lunate surface of acetabulum
non-articular surface of acetabular fossa
head of femur, anatomic neck of femur

fovea capitis
ligamentum teres femoris
transverse acetabular ligament
acetabular notch
acetabular foramen

artery to the head of the femur

medial and lateral retinacula of knee

fibular collateral ligament
anterior superior tibiofibular ligament

pes anserinus

tibial collateral ligament

arcuate ligament
expansion of semimembranosus tendon
lateral meniscus
medial meniscus

posterior cruciate ligament
meniscofemoral ligament

ligamentum patella

prepatellar bursa
infrapatellar bursa
suprapatellar bursa
deep infrapatellar bursa
infrapatellar fat pad

synovium
anterior cruciate ligament
coronary ligament

deltoid ligament
   anterior tibiotalar ligament
    posterior tibiotalar ligament
    tibionavicular ligament
    tibiocalcaneal ligament

plantar calcaneonavicular ligament
interosseous talo-calcaneal ligament
long and short plantar ligaments
anterior talofibular, posterior talofibular ligaments
calcaneofibular ligament

DEFINITIONS

Acetabulum [L., *acetum*, vinegar + *abulum,* a holder or cup]
An early term given to short, wide-mouthed cups, such as those used to hold wine. The resemblance of the hip socket to these is the basis for its name.

Eversion - A turning inside out; a turning outward, as of the foot.

Inversion [L. *inversio; in,* into + *vertere,* to turn]
A turning inward, inside out, upside down, or other reversal of the normal relation of a part.

Labrum [L., *labrum,* a vessel for washing]
Labium, a lip, is used usually to indicate the presence of two lips to a structure; labrum is used for a singular lip.

Ligament [L., From *ligare,* to tie or restrain]

Meniscus (pl. menisci) [Gr. *meniskos,* crescent]
A general term for a crescent-shaped structure of the body.

INDEX

227

228

230

234

239

240